"McGonigal explores the complex picture of chronic pain, recognizing the many dimensions that contribute to one's suffering. In simple, easy-to-follow steps, she takes you on a journey, connecting your mind and body through the yoga experience. This book is very much in line with all that the American Chronic Pain Association teaches. I recommend that you relax, renew yourself, and enjoy your adventure through *Yoga for Pain Relief*."

—Penney Cowan, executive director of the American Chronic Pain Association

"Kelly McGonigal's *Yoga for Pain Relief* is easily one of the best books I have ever read on yoga therapy, and includes plenty of research and practical tips for dealing with pain. This book is perfect for anyone who lives with any kind of physical or emotional pain, as well as for those working with these conditions professionally, including both conventional and alternative health care providers and yoga teachers. The book has heart and soul, is both kind and informative, and recognizes the individual experience without being reductionist or prescriptive. This book will be required reading for all of the students in my yoga therapy training program."

—Molly Lannon Kenny, MS-CCC, founder and director of The Samarya Center, an internationally recognized training institute for yoga and yoga therapy

"*Yoga for Pain Relief* will help you to find your ease, courage, and ability to transform your chronic pain. Unlike many other pain treatments, McGonigal's book illuminates a path free of adverse side effects that is synergistic with your present pain therapy. *Yoga for Pain Relief* is a jewel, and its brilliance and clarity will touch the heart of healing within."

—Julie Good, MD, DABMA, clinical assistant professor of pediatric pain and symptom management at Stanford University

"*Yoga for Pain Relief* is an empowering toolkit for people living with pain or illness."

—Halle Tecco, founder and executive director of Yoga Bear, a nonprofit organization that teaches yoga to cancer patients and survivors

"In this important book, McGonigal elegantly and simply empowers us, through science and ancient practices, to compassionately transform pain and suffering into ever-present joy blossoming in our hearts. A gift for us all!"

—Nischala Joy Devi, international yoga teacher and author of *The Healing Path of Yoga* and *The Secret Power of Yoga*

"*Yoga for Pain Relief* is an epic book for an epic condition. McGonigal is a quintessential teacher and a brilliant author. Highly recommended for healthcare providers, yoga teachers, or anyone in pain."

—Larry Payne, Ph.D., director of the Yoga Therapy Rx Program at Loyola Marymount University and coauthor of *Yoga for Dummies*, *Yoga Rx*, and *The Business of Teaching Yoga*

"Whether you are in pain now or you treat those who are, *Yoga for Pain Relief* will broaden your view of suffering and change your life. McGonigal outlines a clear, step-by-step method, evidence-based yet ancient, to reconnect with the wisdom and joy that is your birthright—the source of wellness that is so much bigger than your pain."

—Amy Weintraub, MFA, E-RYT 500, is founder of LifeForce Yoga Healing Institute and author of *Yoga for Depression*

"In this book, McGonigal provides insightful pathways that can lead those with chronic pain toward a healthier life. Highly recommended for those suffering with chronic pain as well as healthcare practitioners and yoga teachers who work with people in pain."

—Shoosh Lettick Crotzer, director of Mobility Limited and Enhancement, Inc., and author of *Yoga for Fibromyalgia*

"From a place of personal experience, McGonigal reaches out of these pages with clarity, knowledge and warmth. I was not only educated about my pain, but left hopeful that I could come to view it as a beloved teacher. This book not only provides a map for developing a yoga practice through which I can change my relationship to pain, but also empowers me to find my own way via my unique experience."

—Elissa Cobb, director of programs at Phoenix Rising Yoga Therapy and author of *The Forgotten Body*

"*Yoga for Pain Relief* provides accurate, easily understood principles of self-care in a user-friendly format. The book offers professionals immediate activities for clinical adaptation with the best, most up-to-date evidence. The person in pain can celebrate the artful bridging of ancient wisdom with the genius of the author in creating an easy-to-follow, personalized road map that is sure to sustain hope and allow him or her to remember joy!"

—Matthew J. Taylor, PT, Ph.D., RYT, president of the International Association of Yoga Therapists and founder and owner of the Dynamic Systems Rehabilitation Clinic

"Those of us who practice yoga know that it has many benefits, like the reduction of all kinds of pain. Now we have a sourcebook that explains why yoga has this effect. McGonigal's book presents salient research on pain and its causes and explains exactly how yoga helps. This book is a must for yoga teachers and anyone suffering pain. Highly recommended."

—Judith Hanson Lasater, Ph.D., PT, yoga teacher and author of *Yogabody*

"McGonigal's book introduces the healing power of the breath to our society, which is gasping for air. Crucial knowledge for true healing."

—Max Strom, yoga teacher and creator of the DVDs *Learn to Breathe* and *Max Strom Yoga*

"*Yoga for Pain Relief* is a readily accessible and wonderfully supportive manual for self-healing through yoga. McGonigal's extensive knowledge of yoga is conveyed through inspirational stories and practical instructions which demonstrate the power of yoga to transform the mind and body. She has synthesized a wide variety of approaches to 'befriending the body'—combining asana (simple movement), breathing practices, relaxation techniques, meditation, mindfulness, and journaling in very simple, doable practices. Readers will discover there are many ways to work with yoga and feel empowered and inspired to explore and define their personal path to healing."

—Robin Rothenberg, director of Essential Yoga Therapy and The Yoga Barn and author of *The Essential Low Back Program*

"Yoga and meditation are techniques that have proven to be highly useful in helping people relax, reduce stress, and increase well-being. However, it is only recently that they have been applied to the treatment of chronic pain. In this timely, practical, and easy-to-read guide, a number of specific yoga and meditation strategies are presented that can be used by individuals suffering from chronic pain. This book is essential reading for anyone interested in proven remedies for managing pain better and improving quality of life."

—Blake H. Tearnan, Ph.D., consulting and clinical psychologist and author of *10 Simple Solutions to Chronic Pain*

"McGonigal expertly yet simply describes the mind-body connection underpinning the reason yoga is so beneficial to those in pain. She makes yoga more accessible—yes, even to those who thought they could never do it. This book is a must-read for anyone in chronic pain who wants to incorporate yoga into their pain management strategies."

—Dr. Jackie Gardner-Nix, physician at St. Michael's Hospital Pain Clinic and Sunnybrook Hospital's Pain Management Programme, and assistant professor at the University of Toronto, Canada

"McGonigal shares her extensive knowledge and experience in helping people heal themselves with yoga in a way that is thorough and accessible to everyone. May this blessing find its way into the hands of all those who are ready to reclaim their health and vitality."

—Desiree Rumbaugh, creator of the *Yoga to the Rescue* DVD series

"In this excellent and well-researched book, McGonigal provides a lucid explanation of how and why yoga philosophy and practice can transform unhelpful habits into more positive qualities that quell the suffering and stress associated with chronic pain. Yoga for Pain Relief is a light on the path for the millions of people who yearn for methods to relieve pain and live life more joyfully."

—Philippe Goldin, Ph.D., clinical researcher at Stanford University

"McGonigal's *Yoga For Pain Relief* is an outstanding contribution to the growing body of work blending the traditional techniques of hatha yoga with modern medicine. Accessible and inspiring, this book is an invaluable resource for both those dealing with chronic pain and the practitioners that work with them."

—Sandy Blaine, yoga teacher training instructor and author of *Yoga for Computer Users* and *Yoga For Healthy Knees*

# yoga for pain relief

Simple Practices to
Calm Your Mind & Heal
Your Chronic Pain

## Kelly McGonigal, Ph.D.

New Harbinger Publications, Inc.

*Publisher's Note*

Distributed in Canada by Raincoast Books

Copyright © 2009 by Kelly McGonigal
New Harbinger Publications, Inc.
5674 Shattuck Avenue
Oakland, CA 94609
www.newharbinger.com

Cover design by Amy Shoup
Cover and interior photographs by Kim Shetter
Text design by Amy Shoup and Michele Waters-Kermes
Acquired by Jess O'Brien
Edited by Brady Kahn

FSC
**Mixed Sources**
Product group from well-managed
forests and other controlled sources
Cert no. SW-COC-002283
www.fsc.org
© 1996 Forest Stewardship Council

Library of Congress Cataloging-in-Publication Data

McGonigal, Kelly.
 Yoga for pain relief : simple practices to calm your mind and heal your chronic pain / Kelly McGonigal.
   p. cm.
 Includes bibliographical references.
 ISBN-13: 978-1-57224-689-8 (pbk. : alk. paper)
 ISBN-10: 1-57224-689-8 (pbk. : alk. paper)  1. Hatha yoga--Therapeutic use. 2. Pain--Alternative treatment. 3. Mind and body. I. Title.
 RM727.Y64M44 2009
 613.7'046--dc22
                                    2009038431


11    10    09

10   9   8   7   6   5   4   3   2   1

First printing

Any merits and benefits of this work are offered with an open heart to all those who are in pain, with the wish that they find freedom from suffering.

*May you be free from suffering and the causes of suffering.*
*May you know your true health, happiness, and wholeness.*

—Traditional Buddhist meditation

# contents

# Foreword

Yoga may be the most powerful overall system for pain relief ever discovered.

Part of the reason is that yoga is so effective in dealing with stress. Enduring pain can keep your body's stress response system stuck in the "on" position. When you're stressed out, you tend to breathe more quickly and erratically. Muscles tense. Your mood plummets. All of which makes your pain worse.

Doctors typically underestimate the role of stress in causing and worsening chronic pain, and they often don't know how to advise stressed-out patients. Yoga not only regards addressing stress as essential, but has the tools to do it. A number of yoga practices, starting with simple breathing exercises that almost anyone can do, can reliably shift the body from the fight-or-flight stress reaction to relaxation. It is even possible, using yogic tools, to shift your mind and body into a relaxed state when you are in pain.

Also crucial to the yogic perspective on pain relief is understanding the difference between pain and suffering. Pain is the physical (or emotional) hurt, whereas suffering is how our mind reacts to that pain. We imagine the worst. We worry that things will never improve. We decide our life is over. That's suffering, and it often ends up fueling the fires of chronic pain.

Suffering—just like pain itself—can keep the body in a state of stress, which in turn can worsen sleep, promote weight gain, aggravate inflammation, and generally make your underlying physical condition worse. Suffering is a problem most doctors were never taught how to treat in medical school. But the relief of suffering has been a central aim of yoga for thousands of years.

Keep in mind, though, that while powerful, yoga isn't a quick fix. But unlike pain pills, which tend to become less effective over time, yoga becomes more and more effective over weeks, months, and even years of regular practice. The longer and more steadily you practice yoga, the more profound the changes to your body, nervous system, and well-being.

And unlike many other treatments that get labeled complementary and alternative medicine (like vitamins, herbal preparations, or other supplements), a carefully chosen yoga practice is unlikely to interact negatively with any of your other pain treatments, be they conventional or alternative.

In fact, the evidence shows that yoga makes many other treatments more effective than they'd otherwise be. It's not uncommon for yoga practitioners to see their drug doses or number of prescriptions drop. What's more, yoga appears to diminish the side effects of drug therapy, as well as how much those side effects bother you.

Better still, the side effects of a carefully chosen yoga program are almost all positive. Besides its benefits for pain, yoga is likely to make you happier, healthier, stronger, more flexible and relaxed, and more effective in your life.

If you are coming to yoga seeking relief from long-term pain—or are a yoga teacher, a health care professional, or a friend or family member of someone who is in pain—you are in excellent hands with Dr. Kelly McGonigal. Kelly is well-versed both in yoga, based on her years of teaching and practice, and, due to her academic background, in the science behind it. She understands that a combination of different yogic tools is likely to be more effective than any one alone. She also knows that people will differ in which tools appeal to them most, so she offers many choices.

*Yoga for Pain Relief* is a beautifully written, hopeful, and clear guide to a path out of pain and into a more joyful, fulfilling life. May it help you, as the Buddhist blessing goes, be free of suffering and the causes of suffering.

—Timothy McCall, MD
board-certified specialist in internal medicine
medical editor of *Yoga Journal*
author of *Yoga as Medicine: The Yogic Prescription for Health and Healing*

# acknowledgments

I offer my gratitude to:

The entire team at New Harbinger, including Jess O'Brien and Jess Beebe, for reaching out to me, believing in the healing power of yoga, and guiding me through the editorial process.

The photographer, Kim Shetter, for capturing the radiant inner experience of yoga in black and white, and the models, Mercedes Delaney, Brian Kidd, John Rawlings, Jules Skelton, and Omobola Wusu, who are not just photogenic but true yoga role models.

The wonderfully supportive communities at Stanford University, including the psychology department, the Health Improvement Program, and the Stanford Aerobics and Yoga Program, and the warm and collegial professional community of the International Association of Yoga Therapists.

The vibrant and openhearted communities of the Avalon Yoga and Art Center and the Palo Alto Zen Center in Palo Alto, California.

My family, including Brian Kidd, B.B., Jane McGonigal, Judith McGonigal, Kevin McGonigal, Evelyn Wagle, and Herb Wagle.

All my students, who have taught me far more than I can hope to teach them.

My teachers and my teachers' teachers and all who teach yoga in the desire to help others be free of suffering.

# introduction

This book is a guide to ending the physical, mental, and emotional suffering of chronic pain. It is based on the latest advances in mind-body research and the wisdom of the yoga tradition. This book will offer you both a new way of thinking about the causes of your suffering and practical strategies for ending your suffering. You will learn how your past experiences with injury, illness, and other stressful life events have changed the way your mind and body work together. You will also learn how these changes create chronic physical and emotional pain.

Using yoga's toolbox of mind-body healing practices—including breathing, relaxation, movement, and meditation—you will be able to change your experience of pain. As you integrate yoga into your everyday life, your body and mind will become a more comfortable place to be.

This book is for anyone suffering from chronic or recurrent pain. Yoga has proven helpful for all sorts of pain, including back pain, headaches, fibromyalgia, rheumatoid arthritis, chronic fatigue syndrome, carpal tunnel syndrome, irritable bowel syndrome, and premenstrual symptoms, to name just a few.

You may not think that your pain is the worst pain in the world. Maybe you've learned to live with it. But if physical pain is a familiar presence in your life, this book is for you. It will help you relieve whatever pain you have and give you back your energy and enthusiasm for life.

Or perhaps you think, "My pain is the worst in the world, and yoga isn't for people with pain like this." But take heart: yoga may be the *only* thing for pain like this. If you're living with severe chronic pain that medicine has been unable to treat, you already know you have the strength to survive it. Yoga may not cure your pain, but it will help you do more than survive it. Yoga can help you reclaim your life by giving you back a sense of comfort and control over your mind and body, whether or not the pain ever fully goes away.

This book is also for anyone who wants to understand or help someone with chronic pain. If you have a loved one with chronic pain, you can use the ideas and practices in this book to support him or her. Yoga teachers, physical therapists, psychologists, and other healthcare professionals can add a diverse set of tools to their therapeutic toolbox. Each chapter shares not just solutions and strategies but real insight into the nature of chronic pain. The personal stories in this book will give you an appreciation for what it is like to experience chronic pain and ideas for how yoga can be adapted to the specific needs of individuals.

Although this book focuses on chronic physical pain, pain includes not just body aches but also heartaches. As you will learn, these two types of pain are not wholly unrelated experiences. Both modern science and the yoga tradition teach us that there is no clear dividing line between physical pain, such as chronic low back pain, and emotional pain, such as depression. Both forms of pain are in the mind and the body, and both forms of pain respond to a mind-body approach like yoga. You will find that the practices and ideas in this book can also help you deal with anger, anxiety, loneliness, and depression.

# chronic pain is a mind-body experience

There are few things more frustrating to a person with chronic pain than hearing someone say, "Your pain is all in your mind." How many times have you heard something like this and wished that the person saying it could live in your body for just one day—feel what you feel, and know how real your pain is?

But what if these words were actually the key to relieving your suffering?

Chronic pain *is* in your mind—but this does not mean what you think it means. Your experience of pain is real. Your pain has a biological basis. It's just that the source of your pain isn't limited to where you feel it or where you think it is coming from. It isn't just in your shoulder, your back, or your hips. It isn't just a problem of your joints or muscles.

For decades, scientists and doctors thought that pain could be caused only by damage to the structure of the body. They looked for the source of chronic pain in bulging spinal discs, muscle injuries, and infections. More recent research, however, points to a second source of chronic pain: the very real biology of your thoughts, emotions, expectations, and memories. Most chronic pain has its roots in a physical injury or illness, but it is sustained by how that initial trauma changes not just the body but also the mind-body relationship.

Consider some of these recent findings about how the mind and body interact to create the experience of chronic pain, and how mind-body interventions can help:

- For people with chronic low back pain, anger can trigger tension in deep muscles of the back (Burns 2006). This means that your emotions may be as likely to aggravate an old injury as lifting something heavy or overdoing it at the gym. On the other hand, a meditation on forgiveness has been shown to reduce chronic back pain and improve physical function (Carson et al. 2005).

- Physical pain and social pain, such as loneliness or rejection, are detected by the same pain systems of the brain (Eisenberger et al. 2006). The experience of either one can make you more sensitive to the other. This may be why a pain episode makes you feel more socially isolated or why you crave social support when you are in pain. It also may explain why loneliness makes physical pain worse but having a loved one present can reduce pain (Montoya et al. 2004).

- The brain and body have natural pain-suppressing abilities that can keep pain under control. But they typically aren't working well in people with chronic pain. Stress, depression, and anxiety can interfere with these systems, but many mind-body practices can jump-start them. For example, physical exercise can stimulate the release of the brain's natural pain-suppressing chemicals (Dietrich and McDaniel 2004), and meditation can decrease the brain's sensitivity to incoming pain signals from the body (Orme-Johnson et al. 2006).

These findings ask us to reconsider our assumptions about what causes physical pain and how to treat it. They also challenge us to expand our understanding of the mind-body connection.

## Your Mind Is in Your Body

We usually think of the mind as somehow separate from the body. The mind is this mysterious experience we have of being ourselves: it's what we think, how we feel, and our ability to act with conscious intention. But here's the thing: your mind is in your body. Sensations, emotions, thoughts—they all take place in the body. Each feeling, thought, and decision is its own biochemical event in the body, sending neurotransmitters, hormones, and action signals travelling throughout the body.

Sensations, thoughts, and emotions are created and communicated by several systems of the body, including the nervous system, the endocrine system, and the immune system. All of these systems are intimately connected to each other. Together, they compose the biological mind. Their interactions produce your experience of all sensation, thoughts, and emotions—including physical pain—and how they work together will also be the key to ending your pain.

## Why This Is Good News

Finding out that a problem is more complex than you originally thought does not usually come as a pleasant surprise. But the complexity of chronic pain is actually good news.

It means that trying to fix the body with surgeries, pain medications, or physical therapy is not your only hope. If you are like most people with chronic pain, these strictly body-based approaches have helped only minimally or failed miserably. When your physical pain is also connected to what is going on in your mind, trying to fix the body without addressing the mind will never give you full relief.

For many people, the biggest surprise of all is that you don't even need to know what, if anything, is wrong with your body. When the doctors can't tell you what is causing your pain, you don't need to wait for a diagnosis to start healing. Awareness of the way your mind and body work together will give you a more powerful understanding of your pain than any diagnosis you can receive. With this new understanding, the process of healing can begin immediately, with something as simple as a breathing exercise or a meditation (turn to chapter 3 if you want to start right now).

# why yoga

The power of yoga lies in the tradition's deep understanding of the mind-body relationship. Yoga may be marketed in magazines as a way to give you a great physique, but the aim of traditional yoga is to restore health of body and peace of mind.

While yoga has become best known for its challenging physical postures, like the headstand or the lotus pose, you won't see any of those advanced postures in this book. They have little to do with relieving chronic pain.

Instead, you will learn a wide range of yoga practices that reflect the full scope of its healing tools. You will soon discover that if you can breathe, you can do yoga. If you can pay attention to your thoughts and feelings, you can do yoga. If you are willing to explore what the body feels and how to take care of it, you can do yoga. Yoga is not about twisting your body into uncomfortable positions, and you can practice yoga even if you cannot get out of bed.

These simple practices will lead you on the path of ending your own suffering. Yoga can teach you how to focus your mind to change your experience of physical pain. It can teach you how to transform feelings of sadness, frustration, fear, and anger. It can teach you how to listen to your body and take care of your needs so that you can participate in the activities that matter to you. It can give you back the sense of safety, control, and courage that you need to move past your experience of chronic pain.

# what you can expect from this book

We'll begin by exploring a mind-body view of pain that has its roots in the yoga tradition but is supported by a growing body of research in neuroscience, psychology, and medicine.

The central premise of this book is that much of our everyday, chronic suffering is a *learned* mind-body response. Pain starts with a single event, but it is sustained by how injuries, illnesses, and other traumatic events change the mind and body. The mind and body don't just recover from these events—they learn from them. The mind and body usually adapt to previous threats by becoming overprotective. An injury to the back may lead to chronic hypersensitivity of a spinal nerve. A traumatic life experience changes the way the brain processes stress and fear. In the end, these adaptations "warn" you about threats that no longer exist and lead you to overreact to new experiences. This process keeps you in a state of chronic pain, anxiety, or avoidance.

The yoga tradition recognized this process of mind-body learning long before modern science could measure it in the nervous system. In yoga, habits learned from past experiences are called *samskaras*. Yoga philosophy teaches that samskaras are at the root of all unnecessary suffering, and yoga practice is the best way to unlearn them.

This book is devoted to teaching you yoga practices that will help you unlearn habits of suffering and create new healing habits of mind and body. Yoga emphasizes the innate capacity each person has to experience health and joy. Yoga practices are the tools to awaken this capacity and heal your pain.

We begin with the *breath*, which is the central tool of healing in the yoga tradition. You'll learn how to use simple breath awareness to develop a sense of control and safety in any moment, including acute pain. You'll learn feel-good stretches that improve the ease and quality of your breathing in everyday life, and you'll learn specific breathing techniques for dealing with pain.

The next step to healing is *befriending your body*. You'll learn how to listen to your body and develop intuition about what it needs. Yoga practices for making peace with your body will help you overcome the anger, sadness, and frustration that are common responses to chronic pain.

Befriending your body and exploring the breath will prepare you for learning the *physical exercises* of yoga: moving with the breath (*vinyasa*) and holding poses and stretches (*asana*). You'll learn a basic sequence of movements that have been shown to help reduce pain and restore physical health and function. You'll also learn how to create a personal movement practice that meets your needs and is safe for your body.

Next, you'll learn how to experience *deep relaxation*, which is a key to unlearning chronic muscle tension, pain sensitivity, stress, and anxiety. Finally, you'll learn several *meditation* techniques, each targeting a specific aspect of chronic pain, from dealing with pain sensation to transforming difficult emotions. Both relaxation and meditation will help you tap into the body's natural healing responses and the mind's innate capacity to experience joy.

After you've had a chance to try out yoga's healing practices, we'll look at how to make yoga a part of your life. In the last chapter of this book, you'll learn how to develop a protective yoga practice that develops your sense of comfort, strength, courage, and vitality, a "first aid" therapeutic practice for when you are in physical or emotional pain, and strategies for integrating your favorite healing practices of yoga into everyday life.

Within each chapter, you'll be introduced to the stories of people who have used these practices to reduce their chronic pain and suffering. This book also includes a set of sample yoga practices to inspire your personal program, as well as a list of additional resources to help you on your journey to end chronic pain.

## what this book is not

Now that you know what this book is, let me tell you what it is not:

**An exercise program to fix what is wrong with the body.** The practices in this book are designed to help you feel more at home in your body right away. You don't need to fix your body or anything else before you feel a greater sense of comfort, courage, or joy.

**One more thing you will try and be disappointed by.** The yoga practices in this book are supported by scientific research as well as tradition. If you commit to exploring what yoga can offer you, your experience of physical and emotional pain will change.

**Medical advice or an alternative to medicine.** The practices in this book will complement any other treatment program and do not require abandoning Western medicine or anything else that is currently helping. Do whatever supports your well-being and healing, whether it comes from the pages of this book or a physician's prescription pad. The suggestions in this book are not meant to replace or contradict any guidance you are receiving from healthcare professionals.

## taking the first step

You can begin your journey in chapter 1 by learning about the causes of chronic pain. I think you will find that the research described in this chapter can explain a lot about your own experience with chronic pain. It also offers tremendous new hope for ending your suffering. You may even find yourself saying with relief, "Now that I understand chronic pain, I have the power to change it."

If you're tired of thinking about your pain and want to learn more right away about the insights yoga can offer about health and well-being, skip to chapter 2. And if you'd rather have a direct experience of the mind-body connection, go ahead and jump right in with the practices. I encourage you to start with the breathing practices in chapter 3. The breath is the starting point for rediscovering a sense of safety, control, and comfort in your body. It will also be the foundation for all of the physical exercises and meditation practices.

I am filled with gratitude for the practices of yoga and the teachers whose wisdom and compassion have made a true difference in my life. Yoga has given me greater strength, ease, and joy of both body and mind. My own former chronic pain is a pale shadow of what it once was. This is my hope for you.

# Chapter 1

# understanding your pain

This chapter describes a mind-body view of pain that is grounded in the latest advances in neuroscience, psychology, and medicine. This model may challenge some of the beliefs you have about pain, but it will also help you understand many of the mysteries of chronic pain.

## what you need to know about pain

Three important ideas in the last few decades of pain research have enormously advanced our understanding of chronic pain. First came the recognition that pain is a mind-body process, shaped not just by physical injury and illness but also by thoughts, emotions, stress, and learning. The second major realization was that when pain becomes chronic, it no longer plays by the same rules as a typical healthy pain response. The final advancement has been the growing understanding of how to access the mind and body's natural pain-suppressing systems through breathing, relaxation, meditation, or movement.

These three ideas—now commonly accepted in the medical field—help explain both why pain becomes persistent and what you can do about it. Although the modern mind-body view of chronic pain is complex, its complexity makes it rich with opportunities for healing. As you read about the many factors that shape the experience of pain, you can look at each one as an avenue for changing your experience of pain.

## pain is a protective mind-body response

Before we explore why and how the pain system goes awry in chronic pain, let's consider for a moment how helpful the pain system is when it works.

Despite its bad reputation, pain is an elegant example of the mind-body connection. A world without pain would be a dangerous place. Pain lets you know when your physical safety and well-being are at risk. It motivates you to protect yourself when you are being harmed. And it helps you learn to avoid things that could harm you.

How does pain do all these things? It coordinates a mind-body response that directs your attention and energy to the most important task at hand: protecting yourself.

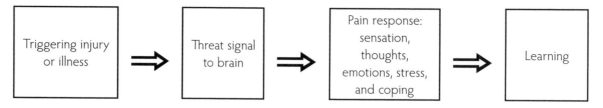

Figure 1. The Protective Pain Response

### Pain Starts with a Threat

The protective pain response begins when the body experiences some physical threat, such as a cut, burn, or inflamed muscle. This threat is detected by specialized nerves in the skin, muscles, joints, and organs that listen for signs that the body is in danger. When all is safe in the world, these threat detectors are quiet. But when there is injury or trauma, they send a threat signal through the spinal cord and up to the brain.

When threat signals arrive in the area of your brain that first receives sensory information, the brain does a kind of appraisal. What's going on? How serious is this? Is this something I need to pay attention to? If the brain decides to pay attention to the incoming signals, the message gets sent to many other areas of the brain that can help you respond to an emergency. This network of brain areas has been called the "pain neuromatrix" (Melzack 2001), but you can think of it like a public address system. The information goes out to just about anyone who might need it or know what to do with it.

This includes the areas of your brain that transform the threat signals into pain sensations, so you know exactly what is happening in the body. The message also gets delivered to the areas of your brain that keep track of goals and conflict. This focuses your attention on what is wrong and gets you problem solving about what you can do to make things better. Emotion-processing areas of the brain also get the message, triggering a wide range of reactions, from fear to anger. These emotions, although not pleasant, play an important role in motivating you to protect yourself. Combined, your thoughts and emotions about the physical sensations of pain make up the *suffering* component of the full pain experience. This feeling that something is wrong is the brain's strategy for making sure you do everything you can to keep yourself safe.

## Super Stress to the Rescue

Thanks to the pain response, you're feeling pretty miserable and motivated to do something to end the pain and suffering. That's where stress comes in. To help you take action, the threat signals have been simultaneously routed to the areas of your brain that help the body launch an emergency stress response.

The emergency stress response coordinates the actions of the nervous system, endocrine system, and immune system—what some researchers have called a "supersystem of stress" (Chapman, Tuckett, and Woo Song 2008). This supersystem rushes in to save the day (or, at least, your life) by triggering a cascade of physiological changes that give you the energy and focus to protect yourself from life-threatening danger. The nervous system increases your sympathetic arousal, revving up your heart rate and blood pressure, heightening your senses, increasing muscle tension, and flooding the body with energy in the form of sugars and fats in your bloodstream. The endocrine system releases adrenaline and other stress hormones into the bloodstream, which further amplifies the effects of the sympathetic nervous system. The immune system gets ready to heal any wounds or fight any toxic invaders by increasing inflammation throughout the body and activating immune cells that protect against infection. These changes can leave you feeling tense, on edge, and vulnerable, but they also prepare the body for quick thinking and action, which is quite helpful in an emergency.

## Learning from the Pain Experience

Even after the threat is gone, the pain response is not over. The mind and body are very interested in making sure you know how to protect yourself from this threat in the future. So the nervous system begins the process of learning from this experience.

If the pain was significant, this usually involves a mental replay of the event long after it is over—recalling the pain, telling people about the pain, analyzing what happened, and thinking about what you could do to avoid similar pain in the future. It can be hard to stop thinking about the pain or worrying about whether it will come back or get worse.

Most people think of this rumination as being separate from the pain response, but it is an important part of the protective process. Pain's imprint on your thoughts and memory helps you learn from your pain experience, making it more likely that you will be motivated and able to avoid a similar threat in the future. Of course, while you're experiencing the intrusive thoughts, it doesn't feel so helpful. But knowing why these thoughts are so hard to shake can help you be less hard on yourself when they come up. Knowing that the mind is spinning tales to keep you safe can also make you less likely to believe the worst-case scenario your mind paints.

The nervous system is also doing its own learning process outside of your conscious awareness. Any kind of injury or illness, even one that is short-lived or appears to be fully healed, can change the way the nervous system processes pain. The body does not just heal an injury or illness but learns from it and uses the experience to predict the future. Every part of the pain system, from threat detectors in the body to neurons in the brain, will adapt in ways that make it easier to detect a similar threat in the future and mount a protective pain response (Tracey and Mantyh 2007).

It is this full set of protective brain responses—from the first pain sensations to problem solving, emotional suffering, stress response, and learning—that creates your personal experience of pain. Far more than just a physical sensation, pain is one of the most complex of human experiences. This is why pain reaches into every aspect of your life, influencing how you think, feel, and act.

All in all, the protective pain response is not a bad system for survival in acute emergencies and handling short-term pain. Unfortunately, the things that make pain so effective at helping us survive in a physically dangerous world are the very things that make chronic pain so complex and so persistent. Let's consider now what happens when the protective pain response turns into chronic pain and what you can do about it.

## acute pain vs. chronic pain

One of the first things to realize about chronic pain is that it does not follow the rules of the typical acute pain response described above. Understanding the difference between acute pain and chronic pain will be critical to your ability to reduce and manage your pain.

Acute pain is an immediate and temporary response to some kind of injury or illness. As described above, it begins with a real threat to the body and leads to a reasonable protective response. Acute pain is, for the most part, a pretty reliable indicator of the threat to your body. If you bump your leg, you will feel immediate pain where you are hurt. If you put your hand on a hot stove, you will feel pain where your skin meets dangerous heat. In general, the intensity of the pain will match the seriousness of the threat—the worse the threat, the worse your pain. When the threat is over and the body is healed, the pain goes away. In short: when you feel acute pain, you can assume that there is a good connection between what you are feeling and what is happening to your body.

Most people, including many people you may have talked to about your pain, think that this is also how chronic pain works. The assumption is, if you have chronic pain, you must have a chronic threat in the body that continues to alert your brain. And if your pain gets worse, it must be because the threat in the body has gotten worse.

With chronic pain, this is rarely the case. Chronic pain differs from acute pain in three important ways. First, the body can become more sensitive to threat, sending threat signals to the brain even when the threat is minor or nonexistent. Second, the brain can become more likely to interpret situations as threatening and sensations as painful, producing pain responses that are out of proportion to any real danger. Finally, with repeated pain experiences, the boundaries between the many aspects of the pain response—sensation, suffering, and stress—get blurred. This allows any one of them to trigger a full-blown protective pain response.

These differences mean that chronic pain is a far less reliable signal about what is happening in your body than acute pain. The pain you feel may reflect a true threat to the body, but just as often, it does not. What it does reflect is a protective mind-body response that has become overprotective. In most cases of chronic pain, the mind and body have learned all too well how to detect the slightest hint of a threat and mount a full protective response in all its glory of pain and suffering.

# chronic pain is a learned overprotective mind-body response

Many forms of chronic pain are best described as misguided learning (Garcia-Larrea and Magnin 2008). The mind and body, in an attempt to protect you from future threats, have learned to amplify your present pain and suffering. Two types of learning play key roles in this process: sensitization to pain and interpreting all threats—even those that have nothing to do with the body—as physical pain.

## Sensitization: When the Body and Mind Listen for Threat

Most people with chronic pain find themselves on guard, waiting for the next pain episode or for their pain to get worse. You may not realize it, but your nervous system is doing the same thing. This is called *pain sensitization*, and it happens at all levels of pain processing. For example, the threat detectors at the end of nerves can become so sensitive that they react to any sign of increased pressure, tension, or inflammation in the body (Staud and Spaeth 2008). The brain, ready and waiting to hear threat signals, can tell the nervous system to prioritize threat signals and "fast-track" them up to the brain (Porreca, Ossipov, and Gebhart 2002). This means the nervous system also gets better at talking about pain, with faster communication of threat signals from body to brain and between areas of the brain. In some forms of chronic pain, even nonharmful physical sensations—such as the light pressure of someone stroking your hand—are interpreted by the nervous system as a threat and can produce surprisingly intense pain (Maihöfner, Handwerker, and Birklein 2006).

Not everyone with chronic pain has all of these changes, but chances are good that some sensitization is contributing to your pain. The important thing to keep in mind is that this kind of learning, and the resulting chronic pain, is an exaggerated response to a real threat. The protective pain response has become overprotective, and the frequency, duration, and intensity of chronic pain can be far beyond any real threat to the body. It can be hard to remember this when you are in pain and convinced that the pain means something is horribly wrong with your body. However, knowing that the intensity of your pain is not always a good indicator of how hurt or sick you are can also bring comfort when you find your worries spiraling out of control.

## Neuroplasticity: Why the Nervous System Gets Better at Pain

Why does past pain make you more sensitive to future pain? You can thank one of the great wonders of our nervous system: its ability to learn in response to experience. This ability is called *neuroplasticity*. Typically, it means that the nervous system gets better at what it's asked to do.

Neuroplasticity is extremely helpful for learning of all forms, including learning a new skill, such as juggling or balancing on one leg. Because the nervous system learns from experience, the brain gets better at making sense of the feedback it gets from the body. It also gets better at telling the body what to do. In the case of balancing on one leg, the nervous system becomes more sensitive to signs that you are in danger of falling. The nervous system also becomes more skilled at using that information to trigger a physical response that will keep you in balance. This is not so different from how the nervous system can "get better" at being in pain. Through the repeated experience of pain, the nervous system gets better at detecting threat and producing the protective pain response (Petersen-Felix and Curatolo 2002). So unfortunately, in the case of chronic pain, the wonder of neuroplasticity turns out not to be so wonderful. Learning from experience and getting "better" at pain paradoxically means more pain, not less.

Keep in mind, however, that neuroplasticity makes any response you practice more likely. This is true not only for the pain-and-stress responses but also for healing responses like relaxation, acceptance, and gratitude. Neuroplasticity provides an explanation for chronic pain but also a solution.

## Chronic Pain and Chronic Stress: Why It All Hurts

Chronic pain doesn't only make you more sensitive to physical pain—it can make you more sensitive to any kind of physical, emotional, or social stress. This increased sensitivity is also thanks to neuroplasticity. Each pain experience that triggers a stress response strengthens the stress response. Repeated pain experience leads to increased sensitivity of the areas of the brain that detect not only pain sensations but all kinds of conflict and threat (Zhuo 2007; Goncalves et al. 2008). This type of learning may play a large role in how chronic physical pain can develop into chronic emotional suffering, including anxiety disorders and depression.

Not only does chronic pain make you more susceptible to chronic stress, but chronic *stress* can make you more sensitive to physical *pain* (Lariviere and Melzack 2000). The physiological changes of the stress response (including inflammation and arousal) provide the perfect learning environment for the mind and body, increasing the chance that pain will become persistent (Finestone, Alfeeli, and Fisher 2008). Chronic stress can therefore lead to the same changes to the nervous system as physical pain experience: threat detectors in the body become more sensitive, the nervous system more eager to pass those threat signals to the brain, and the brain more likely to interpret sensations as painful (Tracey and Mantyh 2007).

If it's getting hard for you to keep pain and stress separate in your mind, guess what: your nervous system has the same trouble. Because pain and stress are both survival systems, and because they so often go together, the nervous system can start to treat all threats—physical, emotional, financial, social, and so on—like physical pain.

Every time you have a pain response, your brain is building links between the many different sensations, thoughts, emotions, and cues in your environment that go along with your experience of pain. When these links are strong, anything your brain associates with physical pain—stress, anger, lack of sleep, the memory of pain, worries about the future, and so on—can trigger a full protective pain response: sensations, suffering, and all. A pain response can even be triggered by threats that have nothing to do with past pain or your body, such as stress at work or a fight with a family member. Even more surprisingly, psychological threats can trigger pain-inducing changes to the body. For example, stress has been found to trigger a unique pattern of muscle tension in people with chronic lower back pain (Glombiewski, Tersek, and Rief 2008). Contrary to the typical pain response, chronic physical pain can start in the brain and work its way to the rest of the body.

The most important take-home point from all of this research is that stress is a big part of chronic pain. It is both a consequence and cause of pain and—for most people—a chronic condition of its own. For this reason, learning how to reduce stress will be one of the most important steps you take in preventing and coping with chronic pain. Many of the things that reduce stress, such as a sense of control, social support, and meditation, will also reduce physical pain. Focusing on these things can be even more effective for chronic pain than trying to figure out what is wrong with the body and how to fix it.

## reasons to be hopeful

Despite what sounds like a heavy dose of bad news about chronic pain, there are two very big reasons to be hopeful.

The first is that your mind and body have built-in healing responses that are just as powerful as their protective pain-and-stress responses. These healing responses include the body's natural pain-suppressing systems, the relaxation response, and positive emotions like joy and gratitude. You can learn to activate these responses to counter the effects of pain and stress and help the body recover from injury and illness.

The second reason for hope is that learning is lifelong, and none of the changes you've learned have to be permanent. Sensitivity to pain and stress can become resilience. Neuroplasticity can be harnessed for healing. Your mind and body have learned how to "do" chronic pain, and your job is to teach it something new.

These two reasons for hope are what the rest of this book is about. You now have a better understanding of the factors contributing to chronic pain, but the most important information is yet to come. You will learn more about each of these healing responses in the chapters that follow, with clear guidance on how to use them to reduce your suffering and heal your pain.

## retraining the mind and body with yoga

The best way to unlearn chronic stress and pain responses is to give the mind and body new, healthier responses to practice. That is exactly what you will learn in this book: yoga practices that teach you how to choose health and well-being.

In chapter 2, you'll learn why yoga is such a promising approach for unlearning chronic pain. In short, yoga is a comprehensive mind-body system that provides tools to address every aspect of the pain response. There are yoga practices for relaxation, reducing stress, dealing with difficult emotions, examining your thoughts and beliefs about pain, and training the mind to be less reactive to painful sensations.

Yoga will teach you how to use your mind as a resource for healing, instead of feeling at the mercy of an unpredictable body. Yoga will also give you a clear way to take care of your body and teach you how to take charge of your experience even when you are in pain.

By helping you transform chronic pain-and-stress responses into "chronic healing" responses of mind and body, yoga will do more than reduce your suffering of chronic pain. It will give you greater strength, courage, and joy in all areas of your life.

# Chapter 2

# yoga: reuniting body, mind, and spirit

While neuroscience, psychology, and medicine are getting better at explaining why and how pain persists, they do not yet have satisfying solutions. Pain medications fail over the long term more often than not. Pain management programs often focus on coping with pain rather than transforming the pain experience.

This is where yoga comes in. The yoga tradition has evolved as a system to end unnecessary suffering. This promise was described as far back as two thousand years ago in the *Yoga Sutras*, one of the first guides to the purpose and practice of yoga.

Yoga philosophy offers hope for freedom from suffering, and its practices provide the tools for healing. This chapter will introduce you to some of the key ideas from the yoga tradition that will guide you on your path to ending unnecessary pain and suffering. These ideas breathe spirit into the science described in chapter 1 and offer a framework for understanding the practices that you will learn in the chapters that follow.

# mind, body, and spirit

Modern science has demonstrated that what we call "the mind" is not separate from what we call "the body." This is a good foundation for a holistic perspective, but it leaves out something essential about what it means to be human: spirit.

Yoga adds this missing aspect. According to the yoga tradition, the human system is not just body and mind but is also breath, wisdom, and joy. Breath is the life force that animates you; wisdom is your inner guide; joy is your connection to something bigger than yourself. Together, these three dimensions capture the idea of spirit. They also point to what is so often missing from a typical medical or scientific perspective: each person's inherent capacity for healing and well-being.

This yogic model of body, mind, and spirit was first described thousands of years ago, but its insights are just as relevant today. Just as the scientific model recognizes that body and mind cannot be separated, the yogic model recognizes that body, mind, and spirit are connected as one whole. All five dimensions—body, mind, breath, wisdom, and joy—are equally important in understanding a person's health. Imbalances in any one of these dimensions can influence all others, and healing that occurs in any one can spread to all others.

## Breath

In the traditional language of yoga, the word for breath and life force is the same: *prana*. Prana is the energy that supports everything you do, think, and feel. It comes from the breath but is animated by the body.

Yogis believe that the flow of prana in your body is what allows the body to heal. When prana is low, you may feel tired, sick, depressed, or in pain. When prana is high, you feel more vibrant, happy, and strong. The flow of prana in your body can be influenced by anything you put into your body—food, drink, medication—as well as anything that you do with your body, including sleep, exercise, and work. However, the most direct link to prana is the simple act of breathing. With this in mind, it is easy to see how the quality of your breathing can influence your well-being.

Because the breath is the foundation for prana, the yoga tradition has developed many breathing practices to support the life force that flows through you. These breathing practices are called *pranayama*, which literally translates into "energy management." This is a good way to think about the breathing practices you will learn in this book. They are tools for supporting your energy, mood, and well-being.

The breath—as it supports prana—is central to every yoga practice you will learn in the book. This is the reason we will start your yoga program with breath awareness and pranayama practices in the next chapter.

## Wisdom

Most of us are used to looking outside of ourselves for guidance. We turn to experts, authorities, doctors, and, yes, even authors. This is fine when you need to gather specialized information or opinions. But the yoga tradition holds that there is an inner guide that transcends the collective wisdom of experts. This inner wisdom can tell you more about what is true for you, and how you can experience peace of mind, than any outside authority could ever know.

In the yogic model of body, mind, and spirit, wisdom is more about intuition and mindfulness than about knowledge or intellect. It is the ability to see what is true in this moment and what is needed in this moment. It is also the ability to see through the habits of the mind—including stress, disappointment, self-criticism, and worry—that create suffering. Yoga teaches that every person has this ability and it is an important part of who you are.

You can develop this ability by paying attention to the inner guidance of your breath, body, thoughts, and emotions. Yoga, and meditation in particular, will teach you how to distinguish between guidance from inner wisdom and unhelpful habits of the mind. Yoga also develops your self-care instinct, helping you understand what your body needs to be healthy and free of pain. When you reconnect to this guidance, you will have a deep source of strength and insight for coping with life's challenges.

## Joy

Yoga identifies joy—a natural sense of well-being, gratitude, and peace—as the deepest aspect of what it means to be human. You might have felt this kind of joy at special moments in your life—the birth of a child, the view of a sunset, or while immersed in hands-on or creative work. These glimpses are not dependent on external events. It is simply easier to be in touch with your natural state of well-being in these special moments.

In the yogic view, joy is the closest to what you might call your true nature. It is not a fast-changing, fast-disappearing happiness that fluctuates according to your thoughts, mood, and present circumstances. In contrast, the ability to feel at peace in this moment is central to who you are. This inner joy is less vulnerable to the changes in your life, and it is not dependent on fixing what is wrong or getting what you want. Even chronic pain cannot take away your ability to feel this part of yourself.

Yoga practice helps you reconnect to this inner joy. Whether it's a meditation on gratitude, a relaxation pose that puts the body and mind at ease, or a breathing exercise that strengthens the flow of energy in your body—they all share the benefit of bringing you back home to your natural sense of well-being.

# samskaras: the seeds of suffering and transformation

If wisdom and joy are as much a part of you as your breath and body, why is it so easy to become disconnected from these natural states? Both modern science and yoga share the same answer to this question: present pain and suffering has its roots in past pain, trauma, stress, loss, and illness.

Chronic pain and suffering are often learned responses based on past experiences. Modern science uses words like *neuroplasticity* to describe the process of learning from past experiences; yoga uses the word *samskara*. Samskaras are the memories of the body and mind that influence how we experience the present moment. Yoga philosophy teaches that every experience you have—including your thoughts, emotions, and sensations—leaves a trace on the body, mind, and spirit. Each experience is stored as a lesson learned about life.

These lessons are not just a record of what you have experienced; they are also a blueprint for how you will react to new experiences. Samskaras become the habits of the body and mind that make you more likely to repeat your past experiences and actions and more likely to interpret the world through the filter of your past experiences. These habits keep you stuck, feeling the same emotions, thinking the same thoughts, and even experiencing the same pain.

## Yoga Is a Process of Positive Transformation

Samskaras do not always lead to suffering—they can also lead to positive change. Just as trauma, illness, pain, and stress leave traces on the body and mind, so do positive experiences. Relaxation, comfort, joyful movement, gratitude, and other positive thoughts and emotions change the body, mind, and spirit. What you practice, you experience. What you practice, you become.

In the *Yoga Sutras*, the yogic sage Patanjali offers the following advice on how to change samskaras: "If you wish to be free of a negative habit of the mind, intentionally practice its opposite" (*vitarka badhane pratipaksha bhavanam*). In other words, if you want to be free of suffering caused by old habits, you need to practice something new.

Yoga is a time-tested system for transforming your habits of body and mind. Yoga practice erases the samskaras that lead to suffering and replaces them with positive new habits of body and mind. Yoga's approach to transforming samskaras is simple and straightforward: one, practice awareness of the habit and how it leads to suffering, and two, practice its opposite and notice if this reduces your suffering.

To take a simple example, imagine you wanted to be free of the pain caused by a learned habit of holding tension in your neck. Yoga would help you do two things: first, to become aware of when and where you hold tension in the body, including the neck, and how the tension leads to discomfort; and second, to learn how to breathe and stretch to relax your neck and let go of the stress that makes you more likely to hold tension in your body.

This process is the basis for every practice in this book. Every yoga practice is an opportunity to leave a new, positive trace on the body, mind, and spirit. You will be guided in how to identify the habits of body and mind that contribute to chronic pain and suffering. You will be guided in how to let go of each habit and consciously practice its healing opposite through breathing, movement, relaxation, or meditation.

## The Tools of Transformation

The yoga tradition has many tools for transformation, and the best way to discover which will work best for you is to explore all of them.

In this book, you will be introduced to a wide range of traditional yoga practices adapted for the special challenges of chronic pain. Together, these practices address every aspect of body, mind, and spirit and will help you rediscover a state of health, wholeness, and happiness.

Let your intuition guide you as you explore the practices in each chapter. When you find a practice that resonates for you, stay with it for a while. Practice it every day. See how it changes your experience of your body. See how it changes your thoughts and emotions. See if it leads to other changes in your life.

Yoga teaches that the five dimensions of human experience—body, breath, mind, wisdom, and joy—are deeply interconnected. To end suffering, you can start anywhere and let the healing work its way through every layer of mind, body, and spirit. A yoga practice that takes the breath as its starting point will influence every system of the body. A meditation that takes the mind as its starting point will give you access to your inner wisdom and help you reconnect to your natural state of joy. A movement practice that takes the body and breath as its starting point can become a moving meditation that calms the mind. Any practice in this book can be the key that unlocks the full healing benefits of yoga.

You can add other yoga practices over time, as you find more and more practices that inspire you and help you manage your pain. Chapter 8 will show you how to put together a personalized set of practices based on what is most healing for you.

# coming home

If you remember one thing from this chapter, I hope it is yoga's assumption that both wisdom and joy are natural, intrinsic aspects of what it means to be human. Wisdom and joy can always be present, no matter what is happening in the mind and body. In this view, wisdom and joy are not simply higher forms of the mind's activity. Your inner wisdom and joy transcend the constant flux of thoughts, emotions, and sensations. They are core aspects of what it means to be human. It is from this perspective that you can say and know, "I am already whole, and already healed, even when pain is present."

Yoga is derived from the Sanskrit word *yug*, which means "union." I like to think of yoga practice as a reunion—an invitation to come home to the experience of your true nature. Whatever is going on in life, you can take refuge in your own mind and body, in this moment, to experience peace.

# Chapter 3

# breath

In the traditional language of yoga, a single word means both breath and energy: *prana*. This is not a coincidence. Each breath, by supplying the body with oxygen, supports everything that you do and everything the body needs. No matter how you are breathing, your breath is already connecting you to life. You can think of every inhalation and every exhalation as a healing act that requires little effort and no prescription.

Your breath is also the part of a stress or pain response that is the easiest to consciously change. There's no easy way to consciously block the transmission of a pain signal from one brain cell to another or ask your adrenal glands to stop releasing stress hormones. You can, however, easily learn to slow down or deepen your breath. It takes little more than a bit of attention to the breath. Small changes in your breathing can lead to big changes in how the mind and body function, including lowering stress hormones and reducing your sensitivity to pain.

The kind of breathing changes that interrupt a stress or pain response don't require learning how to hold your breath or perform any other acrobatics of the respiratory system. These techniques are simple and comfortable, and can be done anywhere, anytime. Research has demonstrated that simply paying attention to the sensations of breathing can reduce stress and make you feel better

(Arch and Craske 2006). The accessibility of the breath makes it the perfect place to begin transforming the chronic pain cycle.

In this chapter, you will learn more about why breathing is such an important tool for relieving pain. You will also learn three different types of yogic breathing practices: (1) breath awareness, (2) freeing the breath through gentle movement and stretching, and (3) breathing techniques for relieving stress and pain.

## breathing is a two-way road between mind and body

What happens to your breath when you are under a lot of stress? When you are in pain? If you've never noticed, begin to pay attention. You will surely find that the breath is one of the first places stress and pain show up.

The yoga tradition has long recognized that your breathing reflects the state of your mind and body. When the body and mind are disturbed by fear, anger, sadness, illness, or pain, the breath becomes disturbed. For some people, pain and stress lead to holding the breath, breathing shallowly, or difficulty with breathing. This is a classic withdrawal response, with the body trying to protect itself from what is painful or stressful. For others, pain and stress lead to rapid breathing and even hyperventilating. This is a classic emergency response, with the body grasping for the energy it thinks it needs to fight or flee a threat. You may find that your own breath follows both patterns, depending on the type of pain and stress.

These changes are a normal and instinctive part of how the body responds to protect you from physical or emotional stress. Normal, of course, doesn't always mean healthy. If you are chronically under stress or in pain, these breathing patterns can become the norm. This is less than ideal, because the same breathing patterns that reflect stress and pain also reinforce stress and pain. They also disconnect you from the natural flow of prana and can interfere with your body's ability to provide you with the energy you need.

It doesn't have to be this way. You can learn to consciously relax your breathing when you are in pain or under stress. When your breathing is relaxed, your nervous system receives the message that you are safe and well. This message ignites a cascade of changes in your body and mind that can prevent or interrupt a full emergency pain-and-stress response. The result is that you immediately feel better, while teaching the mind and body a healthier way to respond to pain and stress.

## using the breath to change your state of mind and body

The two-way connection between how you breathe and how you feel was elegantly demonstrated in a study that observed how the breath naturally changes during joy, anger, sadness, and fear (Philippot, Chapelle, and Blairy 2002). The researchers induced these four emotions in participants and measured the changes in breathing rate, depth, movement, and tension, and other aspects of the breath. They found that there were characteristic changes for each emotion. Joy, for example, was associated with steady, smooth, slow, deep, and relaxed breathing. Sadness, in contrast, was associated with irregular, shallow, and tense breathing interrupted with sighs and tremors.

In a second study, the researchers turned the observations for each emotion into breathing instructions. They had participants change their breathing according to those instructions, with no hint that the breathing patterns were connected to specific emotions. The study found that the breathing patterns reliably created the emotions they were associated with, without any other emotion cue or trigger.

These studies and others like them confirm what you can observe yourself as you try the breathing practices in this chapter. The breath is a powerful tool for breaking the cycle that reinforces chronic pain and stress. When you learn to breathe in a way that supports feelings of comfort, safety, and joy, you can actually choose these experiences over suffering.

---

# THE PRACTICES

## HANDS-ON BREATH AWARENESS

*Notice the movement of the breath in and out of the body and the movement of your body as you breathe.*

*Practice:*

- *Anytime to focus on health, wellness, and the joy of being alive.*

- *During stress or pain episodes to shift attention and to find a sense of safety, control, and greater comfort.*

- *For as little as one minute, or as long as desired.*

You know that you are breathing. But can you *feel* your breath? Do you feel the breath as it enters and exits your body through your nose, mouth, and throat? Can you feel the movement of your belly as you inhale and exhale? Breath awareness is nothing more than this: the practice of noticing how it feels to breathe.

While it sounds simple and possibly not very interesting, the more you pay attention to the breath, the more you will discover. By focusing on the sensations of the breath, you are also learning how to choose which sensations to pay attention to in the body. This skill can be invaluable when you are in pain. While the mind is instinctively drawn to pain sensations, it can be coaxed to pay more attention to other sensations. This makes breath awareness incredibly soothing to the mind and body.

## Getting Started

Breath awareness can be practiced in any position, but you may find that a comfortable seated position is most helpful for keeping you focused. You can sit upright in a chair or cross-legged on the floor, using a cushion under the hips for support.

Breathe naturally with no effort to control the breath, breathe more deeply, or breathe "better" in any way. You're not trying to accomplish anything except awareness, and there is no one right way to breathe. As you become more aware of the breath, you may find that the quality of your breath changes. It might slow down or deepen. It might simply feel easier to breathe. Allow any of this to happen naturally, without any strain or effort to make it happen. If you experience the opposite and find that paying attention to the breath is stressful, you can stop at any time.

The instructions below will invite you to notice specific sensations of breathing. The first time you read these instructions, try each suggestion as you go. Explore what you feel, let your attention rest on that sensation for a few breaths, and move on to another sensation whenever you like. You're getting to know your breath and what it feels like to breathe. This first time through is like perusing a menu and getting to taste a sample of everything before you order.

After this first read-through, however, the best way to practice breath awareness is just to close your eyes and notice what you notice. You will have a sense of the kinds of things you can pay attention to, and you don't need to run down some checklist. Just direct your attention to how it feels to breathe. Let yourself feel the natural flow of energy connecting you to life.

With regular practice, you will find that certain sensations (like your belly expanding or the feeling of the breath entering and exiting the nose) work best to calm your mind and bring you back home to your body. You can then choose to focus only on those sensations when you practice breath awareness.

## Notice How the Breath Moves In and Out of the Body

Begin by noticing each breath as it happens. As you inhale, notice that you are inhaling. As you exhale, notice that you are exhaling. You might say in your mind "inhale, exhale" to stay focused. Continue this until your attention settles comfortably and reliably on the breath.

Now notice if you are breathing through your nose or your mouth. Notice the breath entering and exiting the body, and feel the sensation of the breath moving through your nose, mouth, and throat. Notice if you feel any tension in the throat, jaw, mouth, or face. If you do, invite them to relax. Is there any sound to your breath? If so, is it an external sound (one that others could hear) or an internal sound (one that only you can hear)? If there is a sound, listen to it for a few breaths.

## Notice How the Body Moves with the Breath

Now place your hands on your belly. Notice what is happening as you breathe. Do you feel the belly expand as you inhale and contract as you exhale? Can you feel the movement of the belly through your hands? Can you feel it in the belly itself, as the abdominal muscles and skin stretch on the inhalation and contract on the exhalation?

Next, place your hands on your rib cage and notice how the rib cage moves with the breath. Can you feel the ribs expand and contract? Be patient. Have the idea that you can breathe wherever you place your hands. Let your hands listen for any sensation of movement. Then shift your awareness to the sensations in the rib cage itself. Feel the ribs expand and the muscles and skin stretch as you inhale. Feel them contract and draw in as you exhale.

Now place a hand on your chest and notice how the chest moves with the breath. Can you feel the soft expansion of your chest as you inhale and the fall of the chest as you exhale? Can you feel it both in the palm of your hand and in the chest itself? Notice the sensation of the upper ribs expanding and the lungs expanding inside them.

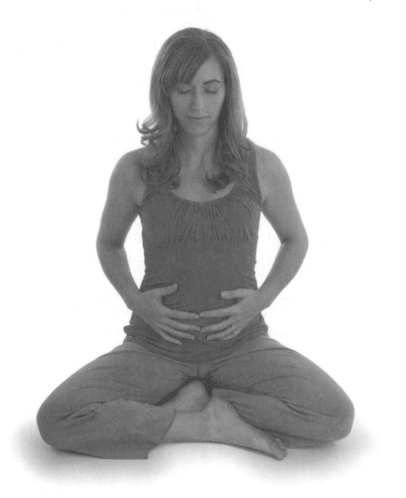

Finally, rest your hands anywhere that is comfortable. Notice the full movement of the breath in and out of the body and the full movement of the body as you breathe. Notice the sensations of each breath in and each breath out. This is your connection to life-sustaining energy. All you need to do is welcome it. By devoting your attention to the breath, you give your body permission to breathe in a way that supports healing and relaxation.

# Christine's Story: Finding Freedom in the Middle of Pain

As a conflict-negotiation and human-resources manager, Christine spent her workday absorbing other people's problems and stress. Exhausted at 6:00 p.m., she returned to what she called "her second shift" at home, where she cared for her aging and increasingly dependent mother-in-law.

Christine had suffered from migraine headaches since she was a teenager, but they seemed to be getting more intense. The migraines felt like a personal assault to Christine. Because the pain was inside her head, it felt both intimate and incredibly invasive. The migraine took up the entire space of her attention, crowding out the ability to do anything at all that required focus. Christine described it "as if the migraine is squeezing me out of my head and taking over." She thought that the pain wouldn't be so bad if it were somewhere else in her body: her arm, her leg, her back—anything that didn't feel so connected to her ability to think and to her sense of self.

What Christine wanted most from yoga was to reclaim a sense of spaciousness and freedom during a headache. Because the pain was literally "in her head," a simple meditation like breath awareness appealed to Christine. She called it "taking my mind back from the headache."

During breath awareness, it was the sensation of the belly moving with the breath that gave Christine a sense of freedom. "It dropped my awareness into my core. I had always felt like the part of me that was 'me' was in my head. When I could focus on the breath moving my belly, I had a sense of self that was centered." The pain did not go away, but she described it like turning down the volume. It was possible to pay attention to something besides the pain.

Christine found that she could also use breath awareness during tense moments at work and at home. It helped her stay centered in the middle of conflict and difficult decisions. She described it as a strategy for not taking in everybody else's chaos and not letting stressful situations steal her energy.

This is what breath awareness does. It can bring you back home to your body and mind and remind you that you are not the pain, the stress, or the suffering that is present right now. The breath can be the anchor that keeps you grounded and safe in a storm. It can also help reconnect you to prana in situations—including pain—that take a lot of energy from you.

The next time you find yourself low in energy, try reconnecting with the practice of breath awareness. Remember that prana already flows through you. You don't need to breathe better or deeper to feel this—just pause for a minute to pay attention.

# FREEING THE BREATH

*Gentle stretches and movements to release tension in the breath.*

*Practice:*

- *Anytime to support healthy breathing habits.*

- *As a stand-alone yoga session or at the beginning of a longer session.*

*A full practice will take five to ten minutes; individual stretches can be done separately for a shorter practice.*

One of the best things you can do for your everyday well-being is learn to breathe with less effort and tension. Tension in the breath can reinforce pain and stress, but a relaxed breath sends a continuous message to your mind and body that you are safe and well. Releasing tension from your breath will let you breathe more deeply and smoothly with no extra effort.

Where does tension in the breath come from? Most of the time, it comes from chronic tension in your body. When you hold tension in the belly, back, chest, shoulders, and neck, the natural action of your breathing muscles and lungs is restricted. When the belly, back, chest, shoulders, and neck are free of unnecessary tension, the natural breath is released.

Gentle stretching is the best way to release the breath. To understand this, think about what it takes to blow up a balloon. When you take a new balloon out of a bag, it hasn't been stretched. If you try to inflate it, you will struggle—there's too much resistance. Even though you are working hard, the balloon does not fully inflate. But if you take a few moments to stretch the balloon out and then try to inflate it, you will find it much easier to expand. The body and breath are the same way: when you release the outer resistance (muscle tension), the breath can "inflate" you with far less effort. Your experience will be of a deeper breath with greater ease.

Freeing the breath takes only a few minutes, but it has a powerful effect on both mind and body. This makes freeing the breath a perfect stand-alone practice to start each morning or as a break at work to let go of the tension that builds up over the day. It is also a wonderful way to begin a longer yoga practice.

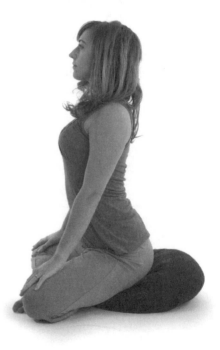

# Getting Started

The following set of simple movements and stretches will help you let go of tension that restricts the breath. The first time you try these stretches, you can use them to discover where you habitually hold tension in your breath. Before and after each stretch, place your hands on your body where the stretch is supposed to release the breath (as shown in the photos). Inhale and exhale in a natural but patient way. Don't try to force a deep breath. Notice whether this area expands and contracts as you breathe. Does it feel fluid with the breath or frozen?

If, after several breaths, you don't feel any movement at all, it is a good sign that you are holding tension in this area. Stretching and gently moving this area will help release the tension, allowing the area to expand when you inhale. After stretching this area, check again to see if there is more movement in this area when you breathe. If so, this is a good exercise for you to practice regularly.

If you don't notice any change, and there is still no movement with the breath, try imagining that this part of the body is relaxing and expanding as you inhale and releasing as you exhale. Imagination is a powerful tool when trying to change the habits of your body or mind, and it requires no force or struggle.

## Opening the Belly and Lower Back

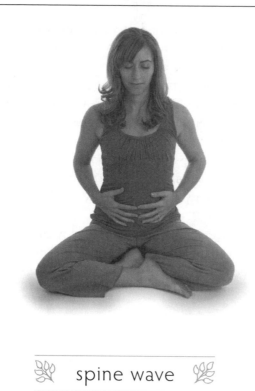

### spine wave

**Releases:** Tension in the belly and back.

**Inhale:** Move into a front-body stretch by drawing your shoulders back to lift your chest and drawing your spine into the body to slightly arch the back. The act of inhaling should make the movement easier and deepen the stretch you feel in the chest and belly.

**Exhale:** Move into a back-body stretch by drawing the chest and belly in to round the spine and stretch the back. The act of exhaling should make the movement easier and deepen the stretch you feel in your back.

What makes this a breath-freeing exercise is not just the two stretches but how you move between them with the breath. Let each inhalation or exhalation begin the movement and draw you into the stretch, and feel the end of the breath complete the movement and deepen the stretch. Find a natural rhythm of moving between the two stretches with your breath.

Repeat for five to ten breath cycles.

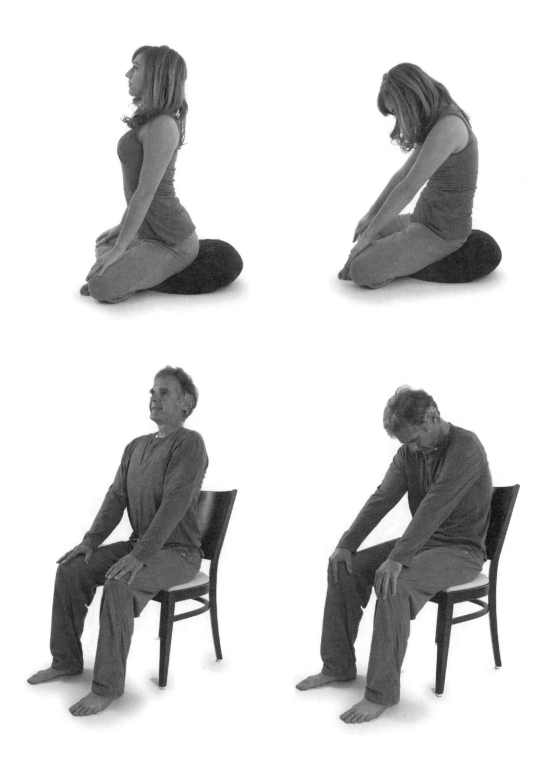

33

## 🌿 seated forward fold 🌿

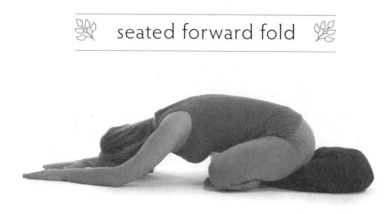

**Releases:** Tension in the back.

Lean forward in a seated position—only as far as is comfortable—and rest on your arms, a pillow, or whatever support is available to lean on. Breathe easily and rest. Feel the movement of breath in your belly and back.

Stay for five to ten breaths.

After the spine wave and forward fold, return to sitting. Bring your hands to your belly and feel it expand as you inhale and contract as you exhale. Enjoy the movement of the breath in the belly and back.

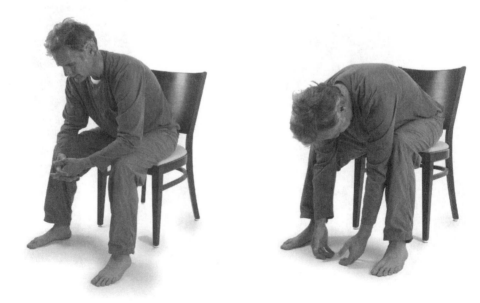

## Opening the Upper Body

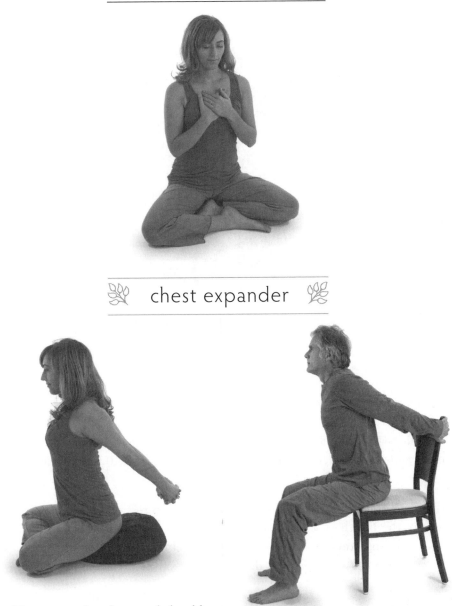

🌿 chest expander 🌿

**Releases:** Tension in the chest and shoulders.

Clasp your hands behind your back or reach behind you to hold on to the back of a chair. Draw your shoulder blades together to open the chest. Find the stretch right where your upper arms meet the chest. Feel the breath in your chest, and let the breath stretch you from the inside out. Imagine the lungs and heart expanding as you inhale.

Stay for five to ten breaths.

## ❧ neck stretch ❧

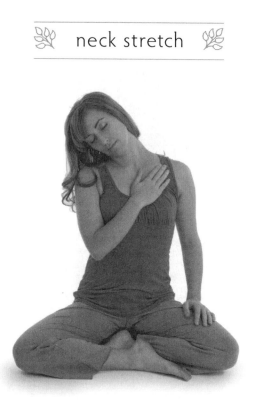

**Releases:** Tension in the neck and shoulders.

Drop one ear toward the shoulder on that side. Bring your hand to rest on your chest, right underneath the collarbone. Feel the subtle movement of the breath under your hand.

Stay for five to ten breaths.

After the chest and neck stretches, bring both hands to rest on your chest. Imagine directing the movement of the breath to your hands. As you inhale, feel the chest expand. As you exhale, feel it drop. Then bring one hand to your belly and feel both the chest and belly expand as you inhale and contract as you exhale. Enjoy the movement of the breath in the front body.

## 🌿 upper back stretch 🌿

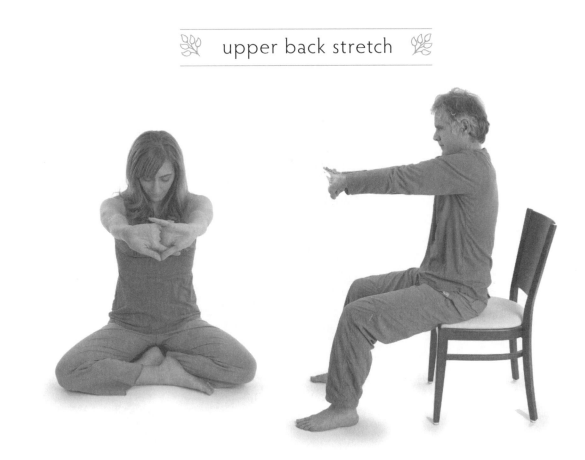

**Releases:** Tension in the upper back and shoulders.

Clasp your hands in front of you. Straighten your arms and press the palms away from you to spread the shoulder blades. Drop your chin toward your chest. Feel the movement of the breath in your upper back. Let the breath stretch you from the inside out. Imagine the lungs expanding right underneath the upper back ribs.

Stay for five to ten breaths.

After stretching the upper back, give yourself a hug, crossing your arms over your chest. Bring your awareness to your back, and imagine directing the movement of the breath to your back. Feel the chest expand underneath your arms. Enjoy the movement of the breath in the chest and back body, feeling both expand as you inhale and contract as you exhale.

## Opening the Side Body

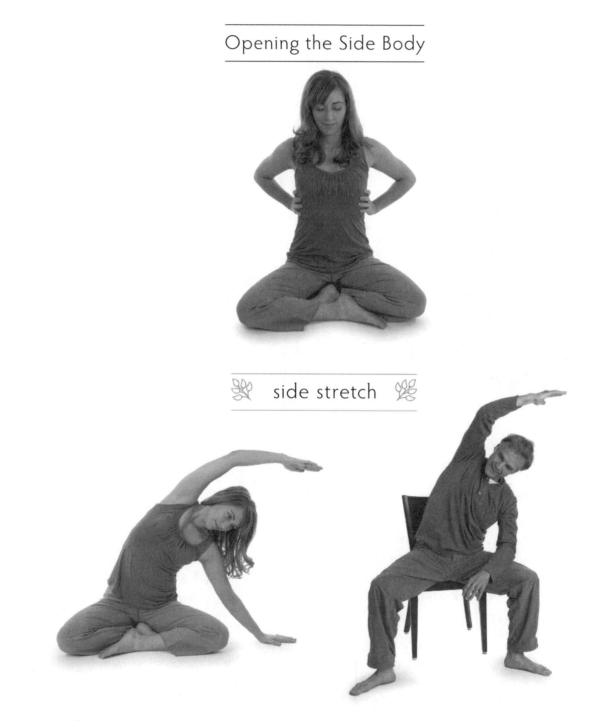

### 🌿 side stretch 🌿

**Releases:** Tension in the muscles of the rib cage and side body.

Lean to one side, letting the spine and rib cage curve until you feel a stretch in your side body. Support yourself on your hand or elbow. Feel the movement of the breath in your side ribs and let the breath stretch you from the inside out.

Stay for five to ten breaths.

After stretching the side body, bring one hand to rest on the side ribs or waist that you just stretched. Imagine directing the movement of the breath to your hand. As you inhale, feel the side body expand. As you exhale, feel it contract. Enjoy the movement of the breath in the side body. Repeat for the second side.

## feel the whole body breathe

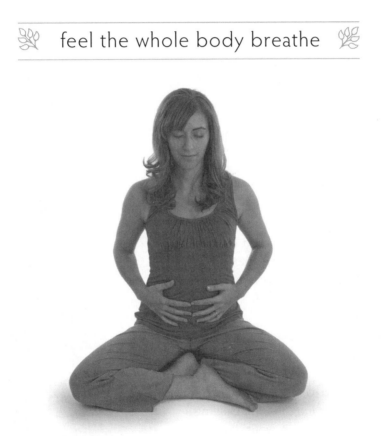

Finish in any comfortable position. Close your eyes and enjoy the sensation of your body moving as you breathe. Notice how the body feels having spent this time stretching and breathing. Did anything about your breathing change from before this practice?

---

# BREATHING PRACTICES FOR PAIN AND STRESS RELIEF

## THE BREATH OF JOY

*Breathe into the belly, rib cage, and chest with a soft smile on your face and the image of your heart expanding.*

*Practice:*

- *Anytime to reconnect to the inner joy that is your true nature.*

- *For ten breaths or as long as is needed and helpful.*

The breath of joy is a simple practice that can change your state of mind by changing the quality of your breath.

Come into a comfortable upright position, seated or standing. Place your hands over your heart, and notice the natural movement of breath under your hands. Relax your face, neck, and shoulders.

As you inhale, feel the breath expand the lower belly, upper belly, rib cage, and chest. Feel each area expand gently, like a wave that starts in the lower belly and crests at your heart. Be patient with each inhalation and keep inviting the breath in (without strain) until you feel comfortably full and radiant with breath. As you exhale, let the breath go without effort. You might even open your mouth and let the exhalation be an easy, soft sigh. Both the inhalation and exhalation should be free of tension. Have the feeling that you are receiving each breath and welcoming it with an open heart. Keep a soft smile on your face.

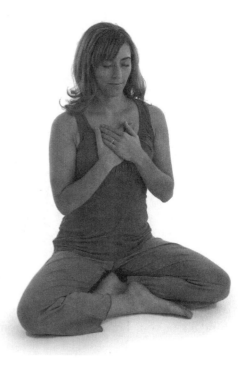

Once you connect to the feeling of the breath, close your eyes. Feel your heart center, right underneath your hands. Visualize one of the following in your heart center: your physical heart, resting between your lungs; a sun, glowing brightly; or a sphere of light in your favorite color. Imagine it expanding as you inhale and contracting as you exhale. Connect to the visual image of it expanding and contracting, as well as to the feeling of it expanding and contracting.

# THE RELIEF BREATH

*Gently extend the length of your breath to a four-count inhalation and eight-count exhalation.*

*Practice:*

- *During pain or stress episodes to find a sense of safety, control, and greater comfort.*

- *As long as is needed and helpful, making sure there is no strain or struggle. Return to relaxed, natural breathing if any discomfort or strain occurs.*

The relief breath can help you get through pain episodes and emotional overload. This breathing technique has helped people find a sense of safety and control during not just chronic pain episodes but also panic attacks, medical procedures, turbulent flights, and just about any kind of stress you can imagine.

The relief breath reduces pain, suffering, and stress in two important ways:

1. By slowing down your breathing and extending your exhalation, it triggers the relaxation response and shuts down the emergency stress response.

2. It focuses the mind on something simple to control. This creates a sense of safety that can make the mind and body less sensitive to threat and pain.

## Intentional Tension as You Exhale, Relaxation as You Inhale

Start by slowing down your exhalation. The easiest way to do this is to breathe out through pursed lips, as if you were holding a straw between your lips. Imagine slowly blowing your breath out through the straw. To keep the exhalation slow and steady, use your abdominal muscles. Pull your belly in as you blow out.

To inhale, close the pursed lips and let go of any tension in the belly. This simple act of relaxation will invite the breath into the body, through the nose, with no effort on your part. Let the inhalation quickly and easily expand the belly.

Continue for several rounds. Aim for an exhalation that feels intentional and complete but without strain and an inhalation that feels relaxed and effortless.

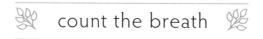

## count the breath

The second step of the relief breath is to make the exhalation longer than the inhalation. Begin to count the length of each inhalation and exhalation. The exhalation may already be slower than the inhalation—for example, you might count to three as you inhale but find that you can count to five as you exhale.

Over several rounds of inhaling and exhaling, move toward slowing the exhalation down to twice as long as the inhalation (for example, inhale for four counts, exhale for eight counts). The key to this technique is not struggling and straining on the exhalation and not gasping for a quick breath on the inhalation. Be patient, and just have the intention to exhale fully. If you strain to lengthen the exhalation, you will create more stress on your system—exactly the opposite of what the relief breath is meant to do. Do not force a 1:2 ratio if it does not feel comfortable. If you can comfortably extend the exhalation only by one count compared to the inhalation, or even just to equal lengths of inhalation and exhalation, that is fine.

After you find a steady rhythm, try inhaling and exhaling through the nose only. If you can maintain a slow steady exhale and easy relaxed inhale with the mouth closed, continue. If not, return to pursed-lip exhalations. During the extended exhalations, imagine letting go of pain, stress, and anything else you don't need.

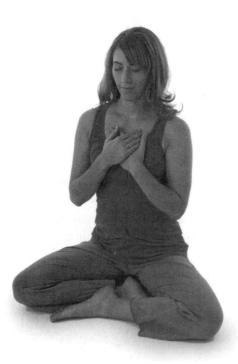

You can continue the relief breath for as long as you like, but often the benefits come from the first couple of minutes of lengthened exhalations. If you find yourself holding your breath or forcing the breath, return to relaxed natural breathing.

For a variation of the relief breath that adds a healing meditation, you can use a yoga *mantra* (a healing phrase) to "count" the inhalation and exhalation. Rather than counting to four and eight, you can use a four-syllable mantra for the inhalation (such as *sa-ta-na-ma* or *om shanti om*), and repeat it twice as your exhale. See chapter 7 for a selection of mantras with their pronunciation and meanings.

# THE BALANCING BREATH

*Part 1 (Alternate Nostril Breathing): Inhale through right nostril, exhale through left nostril. Then inhale left, exhale right. Continue alternating for ten rounds (twenty breaths). Return to relaxed, natural breathing if any discomfort or strain occurs.*

*Part 2 (Visualization): Imagine alternate nostril breathing for ten breaths. Visualize inhaling and exhaling through the right nostril and whole right side of the body for ten breaths. Switch to visualizing inhaling and exhaling through the left nostril and whole left side of the body for ten breaths. Switch back and forth between right and left sides for ten breaths. Breathe through both nostrils, visualizing the breath moving through the whole body, for ten breaths.*

*Practice:*

- *During pain or stress episodes to find a sense of safety, control, and greater comfort.*

- *In bed (part 2 only) to overcome stress or pain-related insomnia.*

The balancing breath is particularly helpful for reducing stress. Its Sanskrit name, *nadi shodana*, literally means "energy cleansing." This is not just yogic legend—research has shown that this breathing technique can wash away the effects of stress, lowering blood pressure and heart rate (Upadhyay Dhungel et al. 2008; Srivastava, Jain, and Singhal 2005). As you practice the balancing breath, you will find that it instills peace of mind and a sense of ease in the body.

## Getting Started

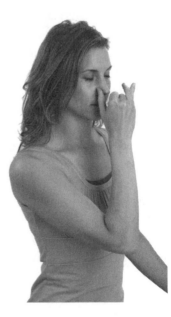

To begin, bring your right hand into position as shown: extend all five fingers, and then fold your pointer and middle fingers in toward the palm. This leaves your thumb, ring, and pinky fingers extended. You will use the thumb to close your right nostril and your ring and pinky fingers to close your left nostril.

Try this now—bring your right hand to your nose, and practice closing the right nostril with your thumb. Notice how you can still breathe through your left nostril. Then release, and practice closing your left nostril with your ring and pinky fingers. Notice how you can still breathe through your right nostril. Keep your mouth closed, and breathe only through the nostrils for the rest of this practice. If this is difficult because of congestion, skip the first part of this practice and practice only part two, the visualization.

## 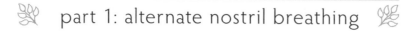 part 1: alternate nostril breathing

Inhale through both nostrils, then close the left nostril and exhale through the right nostril. Inhale through the right nostril, then close the right nostril and exhale through the left nostril. Now inhale through the left nostril, close the left nostril, and exhale through the right. Continue alternating in this way for ten rounds (twenty breaths).

As you practice, try to make each inhalation and exhalation about even in length without straining or forcing. Have a sense of patience with the breath. Allow each inhalation and exhalation to be as slow, steady, and smooth as is comfortable.

After your final exhalation, relax your hands on your lap. Inhale and exhale through both nostrils for several breaths.

## 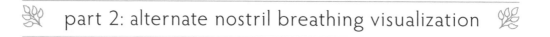 part 2: alternate nostril breathing visualization

For ten breaths, close your eyes and imagine alternate nostril breathing. Keep your hands relaxed in your lap. Imagine inhaling through the right nostril and exhaling left. Imagine inhaling through the left nostril and exhaling right. Continue in this way. Do not worry about whether you are actually breathing in and out through just one nostril. Just connect to the idea and sensation of the flow of breath.

Then, for ten breaths, stay with the right side of the body. Imagine inhaling and exhaling through the right nostril only. As you do this, imagine the breath flowing into and out of the whole right side of the body. As you inhale, imagine the breath flowing into the right side of your core, your right shoulder, arm, and hand; your right hip, leg, and foot. Imagine the breath flowing back out from the whole right side of the body. Connect to the sensation of the whole right side of the body breathing.

Now switch to the left side. For the next ten breaths, imagine inhaling and exhaling through the left nostril only. Imagine the breath flowing into and out of the whole left side of the body. Connect to the sensation of the whole left side of the body breathing.

Finally, for ten breaths, switch back and forth between right and left sides with each breath. For one breath, imagine breathing into and out of the whole right side of the body. For the next breath, imagine breathing into and out of the whole left side of the body. Repeat several more rounds (up to ten breaths), alternating right and left sides.

Finish by inhaling and exhaling through both nostrils and into the whole body. Feel the whole body breathing. Feel the whole body inhale. Feel the whole body exhale.

# BREATHING THE BODY

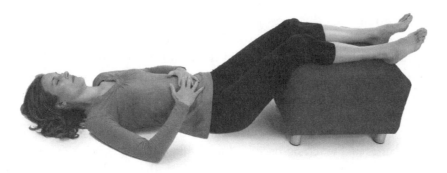

*Imagine that you can inhale and exhale through different parts of your body. Go through the whole body, including any areas that are tense or in pain.*

*Practice:*

- *Anytime to relax or befriend the body.*

- *During pain or stress episodes to find a sense of safety, control, and greater comfort.*

*A full-body practice will take at least five to ten minutes.*

Breathing the body is a visualization practice adapted from the traditional practice of *yoga nidra* (yoga sleep) and the body scan practice taught in Jon Kabat-Zinn's mindfulness-based stress reduction program for people with chronic pain (Kabat-Zinn 1990).

Start in any comfortable relaxation pose, as shown. See chapter 6 for alternative relaxation poses.

Place your hands on your belly and feel the movement of the breath. Notice the belly rising and falling, and notice the breath moving in and out of your body.

In this practice, you will imagine that you can inhale and exhale through different parts of your body—as if your nostrils were moved to that part of the body.

Start with your feet. Imagine that you can inhale and exhale through the soles of your feet. Imagine the breath entering your body through the soles of your feet, and exiting your body through the soles of your feet. Notice any sensations in your feet. Imagine the sensation of breathing through your feet. Feel, or imagine, that flow of energy in the feet as you breathe.

Now repeat this visualization for other parts of your body: Your lower legs, knees, and upper legs. Your hips, lower back, middle back, and upper back. Your belly and chest. Your shoulders, upper arms, elbows, lower arms, hands. Your neck. Your forehead and the crown of your head.

When you get to an area that feels tense, uncomfortable, or painful, don't skip it. There are several things you can try that may make you feel more comfortable.

First, stay with the visualization, and direct the breath right at the sensations of discomfort or pain. Imagine that the breath is dissolving or massaging the tension and pain. Imagine the solidity of the tension or pain softening. Find the space inside the pain.

Second, try moving your attention back and forth between the uncomfortable area and a more comfortable area. For a few breaths, breathe into the painful area; for the next few breaths, breathe into another area. Switching back and forth like this can teach the mind how to give the uncomfortable sensations less priority. You are practicing a healthy kind of distraction: intentional shifting of your focus while still being present in your body.

When you have worked your way through the whole body, let yourself feel the breath enter the body through your nose, mouth, and throat. Imagine the whole body receiving the breath. Feel the whole body breathing. Imagine the sensation of breathing through your whole body, as if the whole body were gently expanding as you inhale and contracting as you exhale. Feel, or imagine, the flow of energy through your whole body.

## Ann's Story: Overcoming Insomnia

Like most people with chronic pain, Ann had trouble sleeping. Her bed was no longer a welcome retreat. Every attempt to fall asleep had become an up-close-and-personal encounter with pain and fear.

At age sixty-two, Ann was almost ready to join her husband in retirement. They planned to spend time traveling and getting in some adventures, like they had done before they had children. To her dismay, though, Ann felt like her body was "breaking down" too soon. Muscle aches and joint pain were a regular part of life, and they got worse (or, as Ann would say, "louder") at night.

Ann would crawl under the covers, close her eyes, and find herself face to face with the physical sensations of pain. Without other sensory stimulation to distract her, the pain sensations had her full attention. She frequently found herself caught in fear, anger, and sadness about her pain. She was kept awake by the thought that her life would get smaller and smaller, and more and more uncomfortable, as she grew older.

The pain and worrying led to insomnia and restless sleep. Ann slept poorly and began to worry during the day about whether she would be able to sleep well that night. She anticipated how tired she would be the next day and found herself saying no to activities and invitations.

Ann's body and mind had learned to associate the act of going to bed with a stress response. As she prepared for sleep, her mind became more vigilant, anticipating pain and anxiety. As she lay in bed, her heart raced and her muscles tensed. This stress response was contributing to both her pain and her insomnia.

Ann needed to retrain her body and mind to view the bed as a safe haven. She also needed tools to shut down the stress response and focus her mind. Ann started this process by trying a few different breathing, relaxation, and meditation practices during the day, outside of bed. It was important for Ann be comfortable with any technique before she applied it to her insomnia. Otherwise, it would be more difficult to learn, and she might even come to associate the technique with the stress she felt at night.

Ann found that the most helpful techniques for calming her busy mind and helping her physically relax were the breathing visualizations. She found the visualizations a pleasant challenge that fully occupied her mind. Once Ann was confident in her ability to relax during the Balancing Breath and Breathing the Body, she tried them in bed before going to sleep. To her delight the next morning, Ann had found it easier to fall asleep, and she was more rested when she woke up.

Ann developed a routine of practicing five minutes of gentle breathing stretches in a chair before going to bed each night, to prepare her for her breath visualizations. She then used the visualization to focus her mind and relax her body as she waited to fall asleep. This ritual helped Ann break free of the pain-stress-insomnia cycle. The aches and pains didn't disappear, but they also didn't keep Ann up at night. With more restful sleep, she had more energy during the day. What Ann had feared most was that pain would get in the way of life, so this outcome was a huge boost to her sense of control and optimism about the future.

If you, like Ann, have trouble falling asleep at night, you can use breathing, relaxation, or meditation practices to make the mind and body feel safe enough to welcome sleep. At first, practice them outside of the bedroom. Once you have confidence in a particular relaxation technique, make it part of your bedtime routine.

## putting it together

As you learn the practices in this book, I encourage you to start putting them together in ways that inspire you. Each of the following chapters will end with suggestions for combining different types of practices to maximize their healing benefits. For now, take a moment to reflect on the practices in this chapter. Which ones appealed to you? Did you get a chance to try each one that you thought might be helpful? Commit to trying at least one to see how it changes your experience of pain.

# Chapter 4

# befriending the body

Kate, a twenty-seven-year-old elementary school teacher, had recently been diagnosed with fibro-myalgia, after a year of unexplained and increasingly disruptive symptoms. She was struggling to maintain her normal life of work and relationships, but it was getting harder and harder to get through a typical day. At night, exhausted but still unable to sleep, she would think about how her body seemed to have turned against her. Would she have to quit teaching? Would she ever be able to find a lasting romantic relationship, when she didn't have the energy to go out and she could barely stand to be touched some days? When the pain was highest and her energy lowest, Kate found herself wishing that she didn't have a body at all. If things got much worse, she wasn't sure life in this body would be worthwhile.

Does this sound familiar to you? Of course, it's not logical to wish that you didn't have a body. But haven't you felt this way sometimes?

If your primary experience of your body is one of pain and suffering, it makes sense that you would want to escape it. When your body seems unpredictable or unreliable, it is natural to feel abandoned or betrayed by your body. You may even start to feel separate from your body—like the "true" you is trying to enjoy life and your body keeps getting in the way. Maybe it's a specific part of your body that you start to disidentify with. There's the true you, and then there's this back or this knee or this headache that insists on hijacking your experience of life.

Many people with chronic pain start to view the body as a prison and fantasize about escaping it. It is at times like this that you might, like Kate, find yourself wishing that you didn't have a body at all. Some people with chronic pain end up in such a battle with their body that they even think about ending their own life. They simply cannot bear to be in this body in this moment and cannot find any way to feel at home in their body.

If you feel this way, it is absolutely crucial that you take steps to befriend your body, pain and all. The meditations and reflections in this chapter will help you do just that.

## what kind of relationship do you have with your body?

How would you describe an enemy? You might say that being around him makes you uncomfortable. When you are forced to be with him, you wish you could get as far away as possible. You feel angry just thinking about him and what he has done to you. You might be shocked and sad at how he has betrayed your trust. You don't want to deal with him. You don't want to listen to him. If you do pay attention to him, it is only because you are on guard, vigilant for any sign that he is going to hurt you. You interpret everything he says and does as more evidence that he cannot be trusted and that he will continue to hurt you.

Does this describe your relationship with your body? Although it can be shocking to realize that you have become enemies with your body, most people with chronic pain feel this way about their body at least some of the time. If you do, you are not alone.

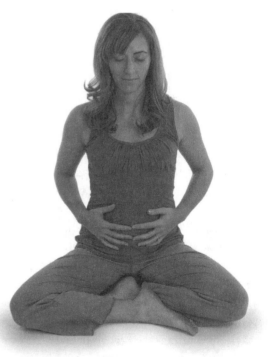

What is the alternative? Consider how you would describe a true friend. For starters, you feel comfortable around her. You feel at home and free to be yourself. Being around her puts you in a better mood. When you've had a bad day or are anxious, you might feel a need to connect with her. You can count on her to be there for you when you need her. You also care about her well-being, and you know that you would be there for her in a time of need. You enjoy helping her. When she has a problem, you listen. You look for ways to make her happy. You encourage her when she's down. You see the good in her, even when she can't. You are grateful for her and can't imagine life without her.

Does this sound like how you feel about your body? Or does it sound hopelessly different from your relationship with your body—so ridiculous that you can't imagine anyone feeling that way about his or her body?

It's not ridiculous, and it is possible. If you're reading this book, there's at least a part of you who is looking after your body with care and support. Take a moment to thank that part of you and invite it to keep reading.

## why anger hurts

Anger, sadness, disappointment, and frustration are natural responses to chronic pain—but natural does not always mean helpful. Negative emotions—including anger—are hooked into the pain system and, for many people, will trigger a pain episode or make existing pain worse. Treating your body like an enemy will deepen every pain-related samskara you have: the stress, the fear, the need to be vigilant to any sign of pain, and the catastrophizing of every new pain episode. Anger gets in the way of your ability to take care of your body and quickly takes over your capacity for joy.

Accepting your body *exactly as it is* will make every step toward healing easier. It will also go a long way in making the present moment, even with pain, more comfortable. The desire to be free of pain and suffering does not require rejecting your body. You cannot walk away from your relationship with your body, no matter how much you feel betrayed by it or want to reject it. As advanced as modern medicine is, it hasn't yet figured out how to trade in a body you no longer want for a new one.

There is a good chance that you will, at some point in the future, be in less pain. But there is no alternative to this life in your body at this moment. If you want to reduce your suffering, you cannot wait until your pain is gone to befriend your body.

## friendliness as a foundation for yoga practice

All of the yoga practices in this book are meant to help you find a way back to viewing your body as a welcoming and safe place to be. Yoga, when practiced with an attitude of self-compassion, will help you reclaim a sense of being at home in your body, even when you are experiencing pain.

I encourage you to set a foundation of friendliness before you begin the yoga movement practices in the chapters that follow. Particularly when you have a history of pain, yoga requires a friendly attitude toward your body. Even in gentle yoga, you will meet physical limitations and experience strong sensations. It takes compassion toward your body to know how to respond skillfully to these challenges. You need to learn how to move your body with both courage and self-care. You don't want to avoid potentially healing movement because you are afraid of getting hurt, but you also don't want to push through discomfort because you are determined not be held back by pain.

For example, you will need to figure out the difference between a sensation that signals real danger—letting you know that you should come out of a stretch—and a sensation that simply lets you know that some kind of change is happening in a stretch. You will not be able to do this if you approach yoga feeling anxious or angry about the limitations of your body. Without first setting a foundation of friendliness toward your body, you may find yourself so frustrated by any limitations or discomfort that you give up and miss out on the healing potential of movement. If you are used to ignoring the sensations of your body, you may find yourself determined to push through any pain you feel, which will only deepen your pain samskara.

It will also be very difficult for you to commit to a yoga practice if you are at war with your body. Befriending your body—and constantly coming back to a sense of compassion, nurturing, support, and gratitude for your body—will inspire you to make time for your yoga practice. You will also find it easier to figure out which yoga practices are most helpful for you. This will guide you as you develop a personal yoga plan that is most healing for your mind and body.

## Taking Steps to Befriend Your Body

The practices that follow will guide you in conscious compassion, gratitude, and acceptance of your body. They are also an invitation to notice how you think about, talk about, listen to, and treat your body in everyday life.

All of these practices ask you to invite in emotions and thoughts about your body that you may not have had for some time. You do not need to, nor should you try to, push out other feelings about your body that may be far more familiar right now. So as you begin these practices, give yourself permission to feel gratitude and sadness, compassion and frustration, forgiveness and anger—all at the same time, if necessary! When negative thoughts and emotions come up, just notice them and continue to consciously invite in thoughts and feelings of gratitude and compassion. This is a good strategy to use, not just in meditation but whenever you find yourself experiencing anger, frustration, or sadness about your body or your pain. With time, you will find the mindset of friendliness more natural, and it will become part of your unconscious, instinctive way of relating to your body.

# THE PRACTICES

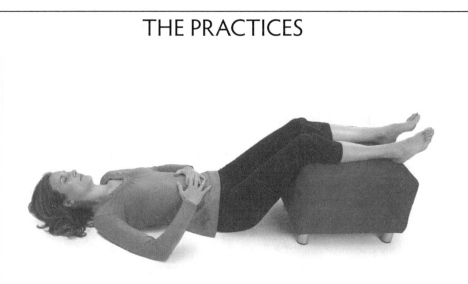

For each of these practices, you can spend time in quiet reflection or write your thoughts out. Make yourself as physically comfortable as possible, whether that means lying on your back with a pillow under the knees, the lights dimmed, and your eyes closed or resting in a supportive armchair with a pen and journal.

# BODY GRATITUDE

*Reflect on different parts of your body with gratitude and appreciation.*

*Practice:*

- *Anytime to repair your relationship with your body.*

- *When you are feeling discouraged by pain or illness, or critical about your body, to consciously choose friendliness toward your body.*

- *After a medical appointment, to remind yourself that your body is more than its symptoms and diagnoses.*

*A full practice will take five to ten minutes, but you can practice the essence of this reflection anytime by simply reminding yourself of one reason you are grateful to your body.*

When was the last time you felt gratitude for your body?

For many people with chronic pain, the very phrase "body gratitude" can seem puzzling, even laughable. Gratitude for what?

You can start with the simple fact that this body is your companion on this life's journey. It deserves to be recognized and appreciated for how it has carried you to this moment and allowed you to experience everything leading up to this moment.

This gratitude practice is an opportunity to reflect on how your body has supported you. Your body is not separate from your courage, your strength, or your journey through life. It is your companion, your home, and the instrument through which your life is expressed. Whatever strengths and experiences you are grateful for you can use to heal your relationship with your body.

To begin this practice, bring yourself into any supported position, seated or lying down. As you become familiar with the restorative yoga poses described in chapter 6, you may decide to practice body gratitude in a gentle yoga pose.

Take a moment to feel your whole body, including any sensations of discomfort or pain. You can take note of these sensations without letting them take over your full attention. Then, notice some part of your body that feels a sensation of comfort or ease. It may be your eyelid, your pinky finger, the soles of your feet, or the belly rising and falling as you breathe. It doesn't matter where that sensation of relaxation and ease is. When you find yourself in touch with that feeling, stay with it for a few moments. Let your attention rest on how that part of the body feels.

Then, one by one, reflect on different parts of your body with gratitude and appreciation. Ask yourself, "How has this part of my body supported me in life? How has it allowed me to engage in life?" Start with an area of the body that feels comfortable in this moment and eventually work your way around the body to an area that typically experiences pain. Some areas to consider are (but are not limited to):

- feet
- legs
- hips
- belly
- back
- chest
- heart

- lungs
- shoulders
- arms
- hands
- throat
- face
- the sense organs: mouth, nose, eyes, ears

Your answers may be literal or symbolic. For example, the heart literally fuels the entire body, moving oxygen to every cell in the body. In this way, the heart supports every action you have ever taken. You might thank your heart for giving you the opportunity to experience each moment of your life. Metaphorically, the heart sings with joy, expands with love, and pounds with excitement. You might feel gratitude to the heart for allowing you to experience each of these emotions. Literally, your feet and legs help you stand and move through life. Thinking symbolically, you might reflect on the times you have stood up for what you believed in or on how far you have come in life.

Trust whatever comes up, even if it seems silly or sentimental. If nothing comes to mind immediately, try focusing on today. What has this area of your body done today? Did it help you prepare and enjoy a meal? Turn the pages of this book? Smile and kiss your dog? Even if today has been so difficult that you have been unable to do much of anything, you are alive. Can you focus on gratitude for your lungs, your heart, and every system of the body that is supporting you right now? Can you feel gratitude for how hard your body is working to support you and give you the opportunity to experience this moment?

Sometimes this meditation brings up sadness along with gratitude, especially if you find yourself thinking about things that your body no longer can do with ease. You may also find yourself feeling critical of some part of your body. Let these emotions and thoughts come and go without grasping on to them or rejecting them. Notice them, as they may be little flashes of the samskaras that shape your everyday experience of your body. Even as they arise out of habit, you can choose to return to the gratitude reflection.

Finish this practice by bringing your awareness back to your breath. Place your hands somewhere on the body where you can feel the movement of your breath. Repeat to yourself, "Thank you for this breath. Thank you for this moment."

## Reflections

What did you notice in this practice? What stood out as something you are grateful for? Was there any part of your body for which it was especially difficult to think of something? How do you feel now? Take a few moments to write down any reflections on this practice, including the things you are most grateful to your body for.

# COMPASSION MEDITATION FOR THE BODY, MIND, AND SPIRIT

*Wish for yourself health, happiness, peace, and freedom from suffering.*

*Practice:*

- *Anytime to repair your relationship with your body.*

- *When you are feeling discouraged by pain or illness, or critical about your body, to consciously choose friendliness toward your body.*

- *After a medical appointment, to remind yourself that your body is more than its symptoms and diagnoses.*

- *Before beginning any form of therapy, movement, exercise, or treatment, to remind yourself of your intention to care for your body and yourself.*

*A full practice will take five to ten minutes, but you can practice the essence of this reflection anytime by simply repeating the phrases of this meditation once.*

In this meditation, you will repeat a set of short phrases offering yourself—and your body—compassion. You can read the statements out loud or repeat them silently in your mind.

In the beginning, you may feel like you are simply repeating the phrases without feeling any authentic friendliness toward yourself or your body. You may even feel internal resistance as you repeat the phrases. Do not worry about this. This meditation can be healing, even if you find yourself experiencing opposite thoughts and feelings at once. You already have the seeds of friendship within you; repeating the phrases is a way to nurture these seeds. In time, the mind and heart will follow the words, and your genuine experience of friendliness will blossom.

To begin, bring yourself into any supported position, seated or lying down, including any of the restorative yoga poses shown in chapter 6.

To connect with your body, place your hands somewhere on your body where you can feel the movement of your breath, such as your belly or chest. As a gesture of compassion, you could instead place your hands on a part of your body that typically experiences pain, if this is comfortable.

This meditation has three stages. First, direct the following wishes toward your body as if it were a dear friend, using the word "you." You may want to direct them toward a specific part of your body that experiences pain.

"May you be healthy."

"May you be happy."

"May you be free of suffering."

"May you know peace."

Repeat this first stage as many times as you like, noticing any thoughts or emotions that come up. Then, direct these same wishes toward yourself—body, mind, and spirit—using the word "I." Take particular care to feel that you are including your body in your sense of self.

"May I be healthy."

"May I be happy."

"May I be free of suffering."

"May I know peace."

If you find it difficult to connect to a genuine feeling of compassion, you might start this practice by bringing to mind a person or animal for whom you do feel an instinctive sense of care and compassion. Direct the wishes to them first, and then let the feeling of compassion carry you into the practice of compassion for yourself.

Finally, acknowledge the freedom you have in this moment to choose health, happiness, and peace, by repeating the following statements:

"In this moment, I am already healthy and whole."

"In this moment, I choose to be happy."

"In this moment, I choose to be free of suffering."

"In this moment, I am at peace with my body, mind, and present experience."

These statements are not positive affirmations or wishful thinking. They are acts of compassion for your body, mind, and spirit. Yoga is the practice of turning away from suffering and toward your innate capacity for health, wisdom, and joy. Whether or not you know or believe these statements to be true, offering them to yourself is a reminder that you have chosen this path.

You may have noticed that some part of your mind wants to argue that you are not already healthy and whole and that you cannot be happy and at peace as long as you have pain. Simply notice these thoughts and emotions and how they make you feel.

With practice, you will find that it is possible to truly rest in your own sincere compassion and well-wishes for yourself, including your body. When that happens, savor the feeling. Let it be an imprint on your mind and body. You can use this meditation anytime, anywhere, to reconnect to that feeling.

## Reflections

How did this meditation make you feel? What emotions and thoughts came up? What did compassion feel like in your body? How does your body feel now? Was it difficult or natural to feel compassion for your body, your pain, and yourself? Take some time to write any reflections on this experience.

# Louisa's Story: Becoming a Caregiver

Louisa, a forty-year-old single mother and legal assistant, didn't just hate her back pain. She hated her back. It's what she said when she talked about her pain and how difficult it made everyday tasks, including work, taking care of her kids, and keeping her home organized. She had always been a perfectionist, and her back pain was making it impossible to meet her own high standards at work and at home.

Sometimes Louisa's frustration turned into a sense of aggression toward her body—the desire to crack her back hard enough to snap her spine in half, and the wish that she could reach her back with her fists to pummel the pain. Even though she knew it was irrational, she believed that her anger would somehow motivate her back to shape up.

When we first met, Louisa didn't have the patience to learn stretches that might relax her back if she approached them gently enough. She wanted to punish her back for causing the pain and was at risk for using even something as potentially helpful as a yoga stretch against her body. Befriending the body was a far more important place to start.

I asked Louisa if she would consider channeling her caregiving instincts toward her back. She was obviously a compassionate, caring mom, but had somehow managed to exclude herself from this compassion. Louisa decided to pay more attention to her bursts of temper against her back pain and to experiment with the idea that her back was something she had been charged with caring for, no matter how it "misbehaved."

Louisa was open to learning the meditations of gratitude and compassion for her body. She found the gratitude meditation for her body difficult, but decided to make it a creative challenge. She assigned herself the task of coming up with one new thing she was grateful for each night before she went to sleep, and she kept a list by her bed. Repeating the phrases of the compassion meditation felt a little forced at first. But she told herself that if it at least interrupted her habit of berating her body, then it was serving its purpose.

With the new approach, Louisa stopped feeling like she was at war with her back. Instead of wanting to punish her body when she felt pain, she learned to use it as a signal to take care of herself. Her aggression toward her back slowly transformed into an attitude of friendliness, which allowed her to play an active role in her healing process.

At this point, Louisa was ready to learn two simple fifteen-minute yoga practices to care for her back: one that focused on strengthening her back and moving her spine (see chapter 5 to learn these movements yourself) and another that included only gentle restorative poses (see chapter 6). Those short practices became a gift that she could offer her back whenever the pain and frustration surfaced.

Consider your own relationship with your body and your pain. Is there any part of your body that you are at war with? What would it look like to take a caregiver's approach instead?

# LISTENING TO YOUR BODY

*Practice:*

- *Anytime to open yourself to the guidance of your inner wisdom and your body.*

- *When you are feeling overwhelmed or confused by pain, stress, or illness, to choose one thing you can consciously do to take care of yourself.*

- *Before beginning any form of therapy, movement, exercise, or treatment, to remind yourself of your intention to care for your body and yourself.*

*A full practice will take five to ten minutes, but you can practice the essence of this reflection anytime by taking a few breaths to center your mind and then asking your body, "What do you need?"*

Pain is not the only important signal from your body, but it sure can be the loudest. When you have chronic pain, listening to your body might seem like the last thing on earth you want to do on purpose—especially if you interpret "listening to your body" as "give all your attention and energy to your pain."

That's not what this practice asks you to do. Listening to your body is about letting all the other messages from your body speak to you—the ones often overshadowed by pain or ignored in your attempt to ignore your pain. Listening to your body is about giving your inner wisdom a chance to offer you some guidance on how to take care of yourself.

This reflection will help you get in touch with the part of you that wants to nurture your body. It also gives your body's wisdom a chance to surface in your open, receptive mind.

Begin this reflection with a few minutes of quiet rest. If you are in pain, rest may not always feel peaceful. That's fine. Just support your body as best you can and allow yourself to feel what is happening right now. If pain is present, allow yourself to notice it. If hunger is present, allow yourself to notice it. If fatigue is present, allow yourself to notice it. This will mark a clear shift from the attitude of just getting your body through the challenges of the day, to a willingness to listen to your body.

Then start the reflection process by asking your body, "What do you need?" Or, if it feels more natural, "What do I need?" Then, ask your body one or more of the following questions:

1. "Is there anything that you need more of that I can give you?"

2. "What do you need a break from?"

3. "What would nourish you best?"

4. "Is there anything I'm doing that you'd like me to do less of?"

5. "What have I been not allowing you to do that you'd like permission to do again?"

6. "Is there anything I should know?"

You might be surprised by what comes up in this reflection. Try not to reject anything. Keep an open mind. Needs that have been ignored or denied have a way of going under cover. They may only be comfortable revealing themselves to a mind that welcomes all thoughts with curiosity and compassion.

Don't worry if the first idea that floats into consciousness seems to have no direct relationship to your body or your health. Take, for example, Kate, the young teacher with fibromyalgia. When she first tried this reflection, the only thing that really grabbed her attention was the sudden notion that her body needed a bedtime story. She ended up listening to classic works of fiction on audio CDs during her worst pain episodes, and it became her most effective therapy. Bedtime stories are not something that any healthcare provider would have thought of prescribing for Kate, and that is the point of this reflection. You are a unique human being with unique needs. As you look within for guidance, you will discover many things you can do that will help you take back some control over your health and your life.

## Steve's Story: Learning to Listen

Years of persistent jaw pain and headaches had taught Steve, a fifty-four-year-old administrator in a university's athletics department, how to function without paying much attention to how his body felt. Sometimes the pain was bad enough to stop him in his tracks, but anything less than incapacitation became like background noise. He had learned to ignore it.

Steve didn't ignore just his pain. He had learned to ignore other signals from his body, like a grumbling stomach asking for food. An uncomfortable back begging for a posture adjustment. The heaviness of sleep deprivation. They all felt like an intrusion.

Steve found that he could operate pretty well without listening to his body's demands. In fact, he began to think of it as a matter of will. His mind was battling his body, and his body was only interested in derailing him from his plans and goals. This was how he had dealt with pain and injuries as an athlete over thirty years ago, and it had served him just fine then.

At first, distraction worked well enough for Steve. But the headaches were becoming more common, the jaw pain more constant, and his pain medication seemed to be getting less effective. A coworker recommended one of my pain- and stress-relief classes at the university. It happened to be held in one of the main athletic facilities on campus, so he showed up.

Steve wasn't really sure what he was looking for or how the class could help. At the time, he had no idea that his headaches were related to how he held tension in his body, how little he slept, and even his tendency to hold on to stress until he blew up in anger. He couldn't notice these things because he simply wasn't paying attention. One of the first things Steve needed to do, to stop the trend toward louder pain signals, was learn to listen.

One day in class I included a "What does your body need?" meditation at the end of our gentle movement session. As Steve later shared with me, this was a real turning point for him. When he first asked his body what it needed, nothing happened. Nothing came up. He was bothered by this and decided to try again the next time he had a headache. This time, Steve was surprised to have a single word come up: "Breathe."

He wasn't sure what exactly that meant—after all, if he weren't already breathing, he would have dropped dead by now. Of course, breath awareness was part of everything we did in class, from movement to relaxation. Steve, however, had ignored that part of the instruction. It seemed less important than focusing on "getting the most" out of every exercise.

Rather than reject the insight, Steve decided to come back to that word every time he had a headache. When his pain flared up, he would tell himself to breathe. Then he would pay attention to how he was breathing. He began to notice that he had a tendency to clench his jaw and hold his breath, especially when he felt the pressure of demands at work and at home. This observation motivated Steve to practice some of the breathing exercises we did in class on his own, to see if it could help or even prevent his pain. To his great surprise, the exercises did help—not just with his headaches and jaw pain but with managing his stress when he felt overloaded and ready to snap.

For Steve, listening to the word "breathe" was the first step to ending the body-mind war he had been fighting. When he started listening to the messages he was getting from his body about how he was handling stress and how he was taking care of himself, he found that he was able to do both more effectively.

The next time you are in pain, why not take the opportunity to ask the simple question, "What do you need?" Write down whatever comes up, and return to it later. Be open to whatever wisdom it might inspire.

## befriending your pain: reflections

Is it possible to befriend not just your body but also your pain? What would it mean to befriend the very thing that you bought this book hoping to get rid of?

As counterintuitive as it may sound, pain acceptance is associated with improvement in pain as well as greater emotional well-being, better physical function, and less interference from pain in everyday life (McCracken and Vowles 2008). Acceptance doesn't mean embracing your pain or identifying yourself only as a person with pain. It means a willingness to experience pain as a part of life, and a willingness to move on with your life even if your pain persists.

There are many ways to explore acceptance as an alternative to anger, frustration, and depression. To start, I invite you to consider two courageous and compassionate acts of befriending your pain: forgiving your pain and seeing your pain as a teacher.

# FORGIVING YOUR PAIN

Pain is a self-protective impulse. As strange as it sounds, chronic pain is usually your mind-body's misguided attempt to protect you from future suffering. If you can recognize the protective instinct at the heart of chronic pain, you can let go of a lot of the toxic anger toward your pain.

Use any or all of the following prompts to write about or simply contemplate your pain and your feelings about it. It is a good idea to devote a few minutes to simple breath awareness or relaxation before you begin, to center your mind. When you ask yourself these questions, don't reject out-of-hand anything surprising that comes up. Welcome all insights and all observations.

1. What might happen to you if you lost all ability to feel pain? Why do you need the ability to feel pain?

_____

_____

2. What is your chronic pain trying to protect you from? What has your pain protected you from?

_____

_____

3. What makes you feel safe? What makes you feel unsafe? Do these things have any effect on your pain?

_____

_____

4. What has your pain given you permission to do or to avoid? Is there anything you need to give yourself permission to do again? Is there anything you need permission to take a break from?

_____

_____

5.  What is your pain afraid of? What is your pain telling you to be afraid of, that you no longer need to be afraid of?

_____

_____

_____

After completing this reflection, acknowledge that however your pain has served you in the past, you are ready to be free of unnecessary pain and suffering. Wish for yourself, "May I be free of this pain" and "May I be free of this suffering."

## SEEING YOUR PAIN AS A TEACHER

Everything in your life—including pain—can be a teacher. This idea is expressed in the Sanskrit yoga verse *guru devo maheshvara*, which can be translated as "Illnesses, accidents, traumas, and losses have the power to bring us from darkness to light."

This verse represents an ideal attitude toward life, but we can be realistic about this: you wouldn't invite pain into your life just to illuminate some great truth about yourself or the world. Still, pain shows up for everyone. You don't have to invite it. When pain shows up, it can drag you into the darkest corners of your mind and spirit. But you can also make a conscious choice to let it lead you to greater clarity and insight. Humans have an extraordinary ability to choose the meaning of their experiences.

The idea that pain can be a *guru*—bringing you from darkness to light—is simply a reminder that everything you experience can make you wiser and stronger. Pain has a way of cutting through bullshit. It can show you very quickly what matters most in your life, and it can force you to take stock of how you have set up your life. Pain can reveal how strong you are. It can shine a flashlight on your fears and your hopes. Pain can teach you patience and courage. It can teach you how to take care of yourself. It can awaken your compassion for yourself and for others.

You can view your past or present pain as a teacher even if you would abandon the teacher in a second. Viewing your pain as a teacher is not a commitment to staying in pain. It is simply a commitment to using everything in your experience—even your pain—to learn how to end unnecessary suffering.

To view your pain as a teacher, consider these questions:

1. How has your perspective on life been influenced by your experience of chronic pain? What feels more or less important now than it did before you were experiencing pain?

2. What have you learned about yourself while trying to live with and treat the pain?

3. What helps you get through a particularly intense pain episode? What have you learned about supporting your own health and well-being?

4. How do your thoughts about your pain contribute to or reduce your suffering? Are there ways of thinking about your pain that make your suffering worse? Are there ways of thinking about your pain that help you find some meaning in the experience?

5. Is there something that you have learned from your experience of chronic pain that you no longer need pain to remind you of?

After completing this reflection, acknowledge that whatever lessons you have learned from your pain, you are ready to be free of unnecessary pain and suffering. Wish for yourself, "May I be free of this pain" and "May I be free of this suffering."

## Jason's Story: Finding the Message in Back and Neck Pain

Jason, a thirty-one-year-old research scientist, suffered from chronic pain in his upper back and neck. He'd had the pain on and off for about two years. Jason described the pain as a constant, exaggerated awareness of his upper back, especially around the right shoulder blade, coupled with regular flare-ups of intense shooting pain up his neck or down his back.

Jason found that the pain, when it was minor, could be ignored or temporarily relieved by exercise or sleep. But at its worst, the pain made it hard to concentrate on anything except the pain.

The pain was also taking an emotional toll. Jason said, "I was disappointed in my body for breaking down. I had taken for granted my body's ability to quickly heal any injuries. This not going away was very frustrating. When I realized the pain might not ever go away, I was just very sad."

This sadness was as upsetting to Jason as the pain, so we decided to work directly with it. We talked about the idea that he could use his pain as a teacher and how that might help him find a little more peace around his pain, even if it never went away completely. I asked Jason to consider the question "What is your pain trying to protect you from?" He answered immediately, "Working too hard." He realized that the pain seemed to be in direct proportion to how much he was working. "Sometimes I'll lose track of time and work fourteen- to sixteen-hour days, and if I do that two or three days in a row, I have pain."

We were both surprised at this response. Jason's original goal had been to lessen his pain so that it wouldn't interfere with his work. He had initially approached the pain as a problem of poor posture and computer ergonomics and went about trying to make work more "comfortable." Only when that didn't work did he consider yoga.

After some reflection, Jason decided, "The pain was calling me to pay attention. It was calling me to be present. To not work. When the pain was at its worst, all I could do was sit. It was asking me to just be, and stop doing."

I asked Jason if he thought that finding a balance between work and the other areas of his life would likely continue to be an issue for him. He agreed that this was likely and that it had been a central issue in his life the entire time he had been experiencing the pain. I asked Jason if this insight changed the way he felt about the pain, especially the fact that it had not gone away quickly. After some reflection, he said, "If the pain is a reminder that I need to find balance, then maybe it is okay if it never totally goes away. At least, as long as I need reminding."

Jason has now taken to heart what he believes the message of his pain to be: sit, be present, and stop doing. He decided to start a formal meditation practice, and he has committed to meditating every day, first thing in the morning. It was the most literal interpretation of his insight that he could think of, and he sees this commitment as a way to test the idea that his pain is related to his work-life balance. So far, this approach seems to be working. His pain is less frequent and less intense. Jason is also making time in his life for volunteering and for music. Before he had felt guilty about spending time in these "recreational" activities, but he now defines them as therapeutic.

Was Jason's pain caused by overworking? Considering how many physical, emotional, and social factors influence pain, that would seem too simplistic an explanation. But even if Jason's work issue is only one part of his pain, focusing on that has helped change his relationship to the pain.

Turning pain into a teacher that you can learn from, instead of an enemy that has power over you, can be incredibly empowering and healing. It can help you find a sense of meaning in what more often feels meaningless, and it can give your inner wisdom an opportunity to help you see the lessons you weren't aware you had learned.

## moving forward with a foundation of friendliness

The practices and reflections in this chapter have prepared you well for developing your own healing yoga practice. As you begin to explore the breathing, movement, relaxation, and meditation practices, remember that each practice is meant to be a gift to your body and mind. Let your willingness to listen to your body guide you in choosing the practices that are most helpful for you. Let your desire to be free of suffering strengthen your resolve to make these practices a part of your everyday life.

## putting it together

Now that you have explored practices for breathing and befriending the body, consider combining two of your favorites into one simple healing practice. This practice can become a daily ritual while you explore the other chapters. Below are some ideas for how to combine some practices you've learned in chapters 3 and 4:

- Combine the Breath of Joy (p. 40) with the Compassion Meditation for the Body, Mind, and Spirit (p. 57).

- Combine Body Gratitude (p. 54) with Breathing the Body (p. 45).

- Practice Hands-on Breath Awareness (p. 26), followed by Listening to Your Body (p. 61).

- When you are in pain, try practicing the Relief Breath (p. 41) for a couple of minutes, followed by a meditation on the following phrases: "May I be free of this pain" and "May I be free of suffering."

# Chapter 5

# moving the body

One of the first things that pain does is freeze the body. Muscles tighten, joints stiffen, and the very idea of physical activity can become overwhelming. When pain is chronic, you can start to feel locked in to a body that has lost its ability to move with ease and strength.

Freezing in response to pain is a natural protective instinct, and many people with chronic pain avoid movement because they are afraid of hurting themselves. But in the long run, avoiding movement usually makes pain worse. Gentle exercise is a far better strategy for protecting yourself from further pain or loss of function. Research shows that the physical exercises of yoga can reduce pain, improve function, and reduce the need for pain medication for types of pain that often make people reluctant to exercise, including chronic low back pain (Sherman et al. 2005), arthritis (Kolasinski et al. 2005), migraine headaches (John et al. 2007), and carpal tunnel syndrome (Garfinkel et al. 1998).

Yoga's approach to movement is a particularly good form of exercise for people in pain. You can go at your own pace, choose the movements that feel best to you, and spend the time needed to learn how to make your body a more comfortable place to be. You won't need to strain, force, or compete to receive yoga's benefits. Yoga is designed to release the energy that already flows through you and to restore your sense of being at home in your body.

To tap into the body's natural healing vitality, the yoga tradition has developed two types of physical exercise: (1) holding the body still in various poses (called *asanas*), and (2) fluidly moving in and out of poses, coordinating the movement with the breath (called *vinyasa*). This chapter will teach you both, using movements and poses demonstrated to help people with chronic pain.

The yoga exercises in this chapter can help you:

- Relax physical tension and stress.

- Improve your mood.

- Release the nervous system's natural pain-suppressing chemicals.

- Regain strength and energy for everyday activities.

- Learn how to listen to your body's signals and take care of yourself.

With regular practice, the exercises in this chapter can free your body from the grip of chronic pain and remind you of the natural joy of movement.

## yoga's approach to moving the body

Vinyasa, or moving the body with the breath, is the foundation of movement in yoga. A simple example of vinyasa is lifting your arms overhead as you inhale and lowering them as you exhale. Why not put this book down and try that movement now? As you inhale, lift your arms. As you exhale, lower them.

The key to finding the *yoga*—that is, the reunion of body, mind, and spirit—in something so simple is to fully unite the movement and the breath. You coordinate the timing of the movement and breathing exactly. As long as you are inhaling, you should still be lifting your arms, and not just holding them up there. And as long as you are still lifting your arms overhead, you should still be inhaling. There is no point in time when you are moving your arms but holding your breath; there is no point in time when you are breathing but not moving. In other words, there is no separation between the movement of your body and the movement of breath in and out of your body.

With this in mind, try the arm-lifting movement again. Spread the movement of your arms out over the entire breath in and the entire breath out. You may need to slow down either the breath or the movement to bring them together.

Did the movement feel different this time? Perhaps more intentional and more meditative? Were your more aware of your breath or your body? As you learn how to fully synchronize movement and breath, even simple movements will become powerful healing meditations.

Asana, or holding poses, is what most people think of when they hear the word "yoga": unusual shapes of the body that are held for anywhere from a few breaths to many minutes. It may seem odd that to free the flow of energy in your body, you would hold still. However, the outer stillness of your body gives you an opportunity to observe the inner flow of energy already present in your body. In yoga, you don't need to generate a lot of energy by running around and getting your heart rate up. Yoga recognizes that the flow of energy is already inside of you, moving through you as breath and sensation. Being still in the poses helps you feel it.

Each pose is also an exercise for your mind. Your goal in each pose is not to go deeper in a stretch or hold a pose longer and longer. Your goal is to experience peace of mind even in poses that create strong sensations of stretch or require effort to hold. As you learn to find peace of mind in each yoga pose, you are also learning how to meet any challenge with patience, courage, and presence.

One of the best ways to make a yoga pose—or any challenging situation—less stressful is to focus on the sensations of breathing, as you learned to do in chapter 3. Breath awareness calms the mind and also helps you stay in touch with how a pose is affecting your body. So for asana as well as vinyasa, breath is once again the key ingredient that makes a yoga practice healing. You will see this principle again as you learn yoga's relaxation and meditation practices. As you learn each new practice, be sure to notice what role breathing plays in it. A consistent focus on the breath will make sure that every practice is infused with healing prana.

## Is Yoga Safe for Your Medical Condition?

Yoga has been shown to be helpful for a wide range of medical conditions, including heart disease, cancer, diabetes, and HIV. Yoga has also been used to assist rehabilitation from surgeries, including hip replacements, knee arthroscopy, and spinal surgeries.

However, that does not mean that every yoga pose or movement is safe for every condition. Major surgeries to a joint can permanently reduce its range of motion, but these limitations vary widely by surgery and individual. Ask your doctor or physical therapist what movements (if any) are contraindicated for your condition. If you have uncontrolled high blood pressure or pressure-related eye disorders such as glaucoma, ask if movements that bring the head below the heart (as in a standing forward fold) are safe for you. If you have osteoporosis or spine injuries, you should be especially gentle in poses that require significant spine movement (as in a reclining twist or rounding the spine to stretch the back).

Unfortunately, there are no universally accepted movement guidelines for specific conditions. But with a doctor's advice and your own willingness to listen to your body's feedback, you can greatly reduce your risk of injury from any form of exercise.

Remember that movement is just one component of a healing yoga practice. Even if some poses are not appropriate for your body, you can still maintain a rich and full yoga practice by including breath, relaxation, and meditation.

# five guidelines for movement that heals, not hurts

Many people with chronic pain have hurt themselves in other forms of exercise and are wary of trying something new, including yoga. Yoga's misleading reputation for requiring a contortionist's flexibility doesn't help the matter. The truth is, any form of exercise can be harmful or healing, depending on how you approach it. The yoga movements in this chapter are accessible to most people. The following guidelines will help you make sure that your yoga practice relieves rather than reinforces your pain. You can apply these guidelines to any form of exercise, to help you stay safe while staying active.

## Balance Effort and Ease

You may have approached other forms of exercise or stretching with an attitude of 100 percent effort—go all out, push yourself to your limits. This approach is more likely to cause chronic pain than cure it, and in yoga, it is a guaranteed one-way ticket to injury.

Instead of pushing to your limits, think about staying in a 50 to 60 percent effort zone. You should be able to breathe smoothly, maintain the integrity of your form, and even put a smile on your face in any yoga movement or pose. Exert yourself just enough to meet the demands of a movement or pose, with the least amount of tension in your body and mind.

If you find yourself holding your breath or straining to breathe, you are pushing harder than you need to. If it feels like you are fighting the pose rather than enjoying it, take the effort down a notch or rest. Try it again with more ease and less strain.

Not only will doing less make the movement safer for your body, but you will actually receive more. Staying at 50 to 60 percent effort will give you the energy and comfort to stay in a pose long enough for it to transform the body's habits and build strength, balance, and flexibility.

## Pay Attention

Yoga movement is healing because it reunites mind and body. Yoga is not something the body can do while the mind is otherwise occupied. Mindfulness—paying attention to what you are doing as you do it and how it feels to do it—unlocks the full benefits of a movement or pose. Mentally disappearing, by contrast, allows you to reinforce old habits, which means reinforcing pain and stress.

As you practice a movement or pose, really pay attention to what you are doing and how it feels. Stay connected to your breath, thoughts, sensations, and emotions. Let your whole body and mind experience the movement and receive its benefits.

This is especially important when a pose creates strong sensations in the body, like the sensation of a deep stretch or the sensation of muscles working to support you. It is tempting to block these sensations out, especially if you have learned to do this with pain. There is a subtle, shifting boundary between pain and the sensations of positive change happening in the body during a yoga pose. If you aren't really paying attention to how a pose feels, safe and healthy sensations can be misinterpreted by the mind as pain. This will trigger a stress response that increases tension and pain. On the other hand, if you ignore sensations that are true warning signs, you are at risk of injuring yourself. However, if you stay curious about sensations and make sure that you aren't pushing yourself, you can learn how to relax into strong but safe sensations while still protecting yourself from injury. In each pose, bring to mind a sense of caring and friendliness toward your body. If a pose is painful, come out of the pose and rest.

## Follow the Law of Karma

In yoga philosophy, *karma* simply means that every action has consequences. This is true for all yoga poses, but the effects of a pose will differ from person to person and even from day to day. To keep your yoga practice healing and not harmful, you need to become a student of karma.

As you practice, notice the effect each movement or pose has on your body. Do you feel comfortable? Are you straining to breathe or breathing easily? Are there any new sensations in the body—and if so, are they painful or pleasant? If you change something about the way you are doing the pose, does it change how the pose feels? After the pose, is there more pain or less? Did the pose increase or release tension in the body?

Being a student of karma also means paying attention to how you feel later in the day and even the following day. Are you in more or less pain? Do you feel more or less stressed? How is your energy? How is your mood? How did you sleep?

As you pay attention to the consequences of your practice, you will learn how to create your most healing practice and avoid poses or movements that are not as helpful for you. This lesson will carry over into other areas of life, helping you listen to your body and care for it with wisdom and compassion.

## Use Your Imagination

One of yoga's great insights into the body-mind connection is the power of imagination. Traditionally, yogis believed that imagining a movement before actually doing it prepared the mind and body for the full benefits of a pose. You can use this principle to make any movement more pain free.

It may sound like wishful thinking, but there's nothing mystical or silly about it. Scientific research has now confirmed that imagining a movement prepares the body to move with greater ease, comfort, and skill. When you imagine a movement, you activate the same areas of the brain and pathways of the nervous system needed for that specific movement. Even your muscles are

## Staying Safe: Sensations to Watch

Safe yoga can produce a wide range of interesting and new sensations: the slowly melting tension of a good stretch; the awakening of muscles you never knew you had; the feeling of your breath reaching into places you never knew you could breathe. Sensations help you learn about your body, and watching the sensations in your body can become a healing meditation in its own right.

There are some sensations, however, that signal it's time to come out of a pose and possibly avoid it in the future. Come out of the pose and rest if you feel any of the following sensations:

- Discomfort that increases as you hold a stretch. Stretches—if you do not push in them—should get more, not less, comfortable as you hold them.

- Discomfort that increases from one yoga session to the next—for example, a pose that felt fine yesterday feels uncomfortable today. This suggests you may have overdone it, and your body needs a rest.

primed to work or relax as needed. Imagining a movement while you are relaxed will also prevent unnecessary stress, physical tension, and discomfort during the actual movement. Imagining a typically painful movement as pain-free can even train the brain to experience it as less painful.

Before trying a new movement, read the instructions, look at the photos, and visualize it in action. Then close your eyes and imagine how it would feel to do the movement with grace and ease. If you find any movement or pose uncomfortable, you can always close your eyes and imagine practicing it, pain free and coordinated with your breathing. Even if you do not practice the pose with your body, you will be creating real healing pathways in the mind and body. You can also apply the yogic technique of imagination to any movement, from getting out of bed to riding your bike, and to any upcoming situation that you are worried about, from a medical procedure to public speaking. Imagining the movement or situation while maintaining a relaxed body and breath will go a long way in helping you cope with the challenge when you face it.

## Be Consistent but Not Rigid

Don't make yoga so complicated or time consuming that you have to force yourself to do it. Doing a little bit of movement every day is better than doing one hour once a week. Doing a few minutes several times throughout the day is even better. If you take the attitude that you need to practice the entire sequence described in this chapter each time you practice, or spend a certain amount of time on your yoga every day, you will set up an unnecessary barrier to doing yoga.

The most important thing is to make yoga a regular part of your life. You want to create a habit of being in your body, and with your body, in a healing way. To help this habit take root, look for five to ten minutes here and there to move your body, breathe, stretch, and relax. The sequence in this chapter is not a fixed prescription. It does not need to be done in the order presented, in its entirety, or for any set length of time. You can choose just one or two movements or poses and let them be a stand-alone practice. Any of the poses can be paired with a favorite breathing, meditation, or relaxation practice to create your own mini-healing practice. See chapter 8 for more guidance on creating shorter practices that fit your life.

## Greg's Story: Doing Less to Receive More

Greg, an office manager in his early forties, had a love-hate relationship with exercise. He was a classic weekend warrior, overdoing it on the basketball court or hiking trail on Sunday and waking up Monday barely able to get out of bed. He would then spend the rest of the week recovering instead of making it to the gym. Two decades of this approach had left him with persistent knee pain and back pain. While he still loved being active, he was starting to dread Monday. It took both a competitive streak and over-the-counter pain medication to keep Greg going on the weekends.

Greg's doctor recommended yoga as a gentler way to stay in shape and reduce his knee and back pain. Greg decided to try a class at a local yoga studio that advertised itself as yoga for athletes. It wasn't the gentle class he was expecting. The room was heated to almost 100 degrees, and the instructor ran the class like boot camp. Greg followed the instructions and pushed himself as hard as he could in every pose. He couldn't help but notice how much more flexible the other students were, which inspired him to push even harder. At the end of class, Greg felt exhausted but exhilarated, just like after a great game of basketball.

Unfortunately, the next day, Greg could barely walk. While he had miraculously been able to touch his toes in the heated yoga class, now he could barely bend to reach his knees. So although Greg had enjoyed the class, he was struck with a dilemma: was yoga just more of the same, or something that would someday heal his pain if he kept doing it?

To Greg's credit, he didn't give up, nor did he go back for more yoga boot camp. He tried a couple of other yoga classes and found a beginner's class that encouraged students to go at their own pace and modify poses as needed. There was no sense of competition. The instructor reminded the class to breathe and to relax unnecessary tension. Greg didn't feel a rush from the class, but after class, he felt good. The next day, he felt even better. He

- Any kind of discomfort or effort that makes it impossible to breathe smoothly and deeply. This suggests that either you are working too hard or your body is having a stress response to the intensity of this pose. The best strategy here is do less to receive more.

- Any kind of pain that is sharp or shooting.

- Any loss of sensation.

All of these sensations are more consistent with injury than the positive changes you want from your yoga practice. You may be forcing the pose or staying too long in the pose, or this pose just may not be healing for you at this point in time.

Use your judgment with other sensations, knowing that yoga is meant to feel good while you are doing it, not at some point in the future. If any yoga practice makes you feel worse, not better, let it go and find a different practice that works for you.

was less stiff when he got out of bed, and he was able to sit at his office desk without the usual pain creeping into his back and neck.

After a few more weekly classes, Greg was convinced that yoga worked. He took some of the most basic movements from the class and started a mini routine at home in his living room. Almost every day after work, he practiced for about fifteen minutes. He was patient in the stretches that challenged him the most. This short daily routine was enough to spread the benefits of yoga throughout the week. He felt lighter, looser, and more at ease in his body.

Originally, Greg had hoped that yoga would help him maintain his weekend warrior status. To his surprise, he found himself taking a more balanced approach to exercise. Because he wasn't in as much pain during the week, he was able to go to the office gym for a light workout during his lunch break. And on the weekends, he became more aware of his energy and the signs that he was reaching his limits. He learned how not to push his body so far that he'd be back in pain on Monday.

Greg is a good example of how to approach your own yoga practice. It can be tempting to approach yoga with an attitude that makes your pain worse. Competitiveness, self-criticism, anxiety, fear, avoidance, and impatience can all derail your best intentions. To make sure that your own approach to yoga is healing, keep in mind that the experience you have during your practice is a good indicator of what long-term benefits you will see. If the practice is stressful, it will not reduce your stress. If the practice is painful, it will not relieve your pain. But if you can stay mentally relaxed and physically comfortable even while moving and stretching the body, you are well on your way to taking that feeling into the rest of your life. Whether you stick with the sequence in this book or branch out to DVDs and classes, let your body tell you what works for you. And when you find something that makes you feel better, make it a part of your life.

# THE SEQUENCE

The sequence that follows is a basic, well-rounded practice that includes poses and movements that have been demonstrated to help people with chronic pain. The sequence is organized into six pairs of active poses and one set of three gentle poses to prepare you for relaxation. Each pair of active poses represents both a vinyasa (a continuous flow between the two poses) and poses you could also practice separately.

An excellent way to practice the active poses in this sequence is to approach each pair as a flow first, moving between the two poses with each breath. Then hold each pose for five to ten breaths before moving on to the next pair of poses. Always rest for a few breaths between poses and flows. Use this time to observe the effects of the movement on your body, mind, and spirit. This approach maximizes the healing power of the sequence. The final three gentle poses can be held for five to ten breaths or even longer. Rest in these poses rather than trying to work at them. Allow each pose to unwind any lingering tension in the body and breath.

Each pose will include guidelines for action—what to do—as well as sensation, or what to notice and feel. The action guidelines help to make sure the movement is safe. Follow the instructions for each pose as best you can. Then let your experience in the pose—are you comfortable? in pain? enjoying the pose?—be your primary source of feedback about whether you're doing the pose right. Sensation and breath will give you the best feedback about whether a pose is safe and healing for you.

One of the clearest signs that a pose is not right for you (at least for now) is when you experience strong uncomfortable sensations that make it difficult to pay attention to the breath and the other sensations listed for each pose. When this happens, try to modify the pose until it is comfortable enough that you can pay attention to the breath and other recommended sensations. If your experience in the pose is still dominated by sensations of pain or strain, come out of the pose, rest, and try another sequence.

You can practice this sequence in the order it is presented or build a shorter practice based on your needs. Chapter 8 contains sample individualized practices as well as guidelines for designing your own personal practice.

For each sequence, modified versions using a chair for support are also shown. These chair versions offer the same benefits as the basic sequence but may be more enjoyable if you are looking for a practice that is gentle on the joints and provides extra support for balance and strength. You may also find the chair versions to be a great way to bring yoga into places where it would be impractical to roll out a mat and get on the floor. Simple chair yoga poses can be a great break at the office, in waiting rooms, and even at the airport. (Ignore any funny looks you get—the benefits from an impromptu yoga session are worth being a public role model for yoga!)

## What You Need

A yoga mat (called a "sticky mat" because it prevents slipping) is helpful but not necessary. You can practice on another type of exercise mat, a hard floor, or a carpet, as long as you feel supported. A mat, towel, or blanket for the floor poses will make you more comfortable. You may want a sturdy chair nearby to try some of the chair variations. If you're interested in buying a yoga mat or blankets and cushions designed especially for yoga practice, see the resources section at the end of this book.

## What You Don't Need

If possible, practice barefoot. Take off any jewelry, watches, or restrictive clothing that will interfere with your comfort or breathing. I also recommend not practicing in front of a mirror on a regular basis. While it can be helpful to get some visual feedback when you are first learning poses, mirrors can take you right out of your body's experience and into self-criticism or distraction. Better to feel the poses, from the inside out, than spend your energy evaluating what you look like in them.

# SUN BREATH
# (MOUNTAIN POSE AND SUN POSE)

These poses connect you to the flow of breath and energy in your body.

**Start in:** Mountain pose

**Inhale:** Sun pose

**Exhale:** Mountain pose

## 🌿 mountain pose 🌿

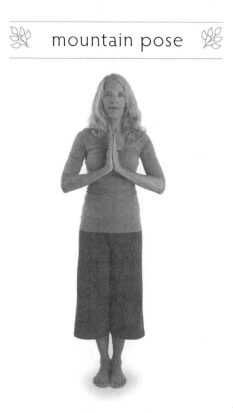

Mountain pose is an opportunity to explore pain-free posture and embody calm confidence.

**Do:** Stand with your feet together or hips-distance apart. Explore how it feels to stand and find your most comfortable stance. When you feel steady and balanced, bring your hands together in front of your chest. Close your eyes or gaze at your hands.

**Feel:** The grounding of both feet, the symmetry of your body, and the movement of breath where your hands join your heart.

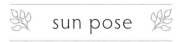

## sun pose

Sun pose is a gesture of radiant joy that naturally deepens the breath.

**Do**: Lift your arms overhead, stretch your hands and fingers, and gently look up.

**Feel**: The length and lift of your upper body and the movement of breath in your belly and rib cage.

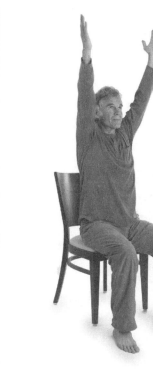

# THE YOGA WARRIOR
## (PEACEFUL WARRIOR POSE AND COURAGEOUS WARRIOR POSE)

The warrior poses strengthen the body while helping you connect to inner strength and peace.

**Start in:** Peaceful warrior pose

**Inhale:** Courageous warrior pose

**Exhale:** Peaceful warrior pose

## peaceful warrior pose

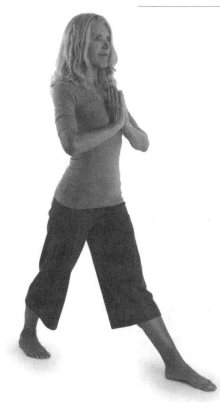

Peaceful warrior is an opportunity to practice relaxing into breath and sensation, without having to do anything or change anything.

Do: Stand with one foot ahead of the other and far enough apart to come into a comfortable lunge (for courageous warrior). Test this by bending your front knee. Make sure that the front knee stops right over the front heel, not all the way over the toes. Then relax back into a resting stance, both legs straight, with your hands at your heart. Close your eyes or gaze at your hands.

Feel: The strength and steadiness of your legs, the relaxation of your face, and the movement of breath where your hands join your heart.

## 🌿 courageous warrior pose 🌿

Courageous warrior brings energy to the whole body and is an opportunity to connect to the feeling of meeting life with an open heart and willing spirit.

**Do**: Bend the front knee and lift your arms overhead, keeping the shoulders and neck relaxed. Gently look up. As you stretch your arms and hands up, ground down through both feet as if rooting into the earth.

**Feel**: The commitment of both legs, strong and grounded; the movement of the breath in your belly, ribs, and chest; and a sense of the whole body radiant with energy.

# STRENGTH AND SURRENDER
## (FIERCE POSE AND FORWARD FOLD)

This sequence strengthens and stretches the whole body, while exploring two very different ways of meeting a challenge: commitment and letting go.

**Start in:** Mountain pose

**Inhale:** Fierce pose

**Exhale:** Forward fold

**Optional Step:** Return to mountain pose after each cycle to rest for one breath.

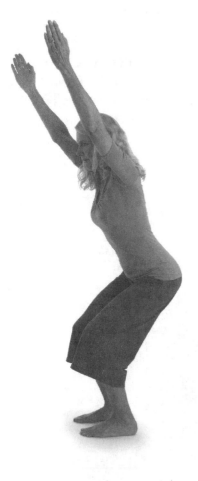

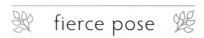
### fierce pose

Fierce pose strengthens the lower body and core and provides an opportunity to practice peace of mind and steadiness in a difficult situation.

**Do:** Bend your knees, sit your hips back, and lean the torso forward. Lift your arms and keep the spine as straight as possible. Remember to breathe.

**Feel:** Notice the sensations of effort in this pose, which can be quite challenging to hold. Be curious about how the sensations of effort and strength differ from the sensations of pain and exhaustion. Can you stay in this pose with strength and commitment but not extreme discomfort?

## 🌿 forward fold 🌿

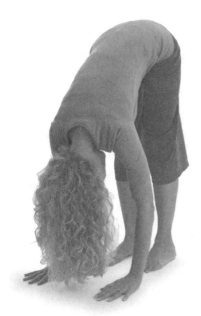

Forward fold releases tension in the arms, shoulders, neck, back, hips, and legs, and is an opportunity to practice letting go of unnecessary physical or mental stress.

**Do:** With slightly bent knees, fold forward from the hips. Relax your back and upper body and let gravity draw you into the pose. It doesn't matter how far you go, as long as you are comfortable.

**Feel:** The sensation of stretch in your back, hips, and legs and the sense of relaxed heaviness in your upper body. How does the sensation of stretch differ from pain? Can you relax into the sensation and stay in this pose without doing anything except letting go?

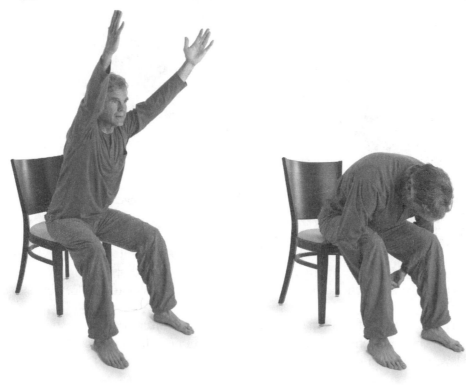

# BOWING IN GRATITUDE
## (DOWNWARD-FACING DOG POSE AND CHILD'S POSE)

This sequence takes two of the best full-body stretches in all of yoga and links them together to express reverence and gratitude for each breath and each moment.

This flow uses a new breathing pattern that slows down the transition between poses. Always move between the two poses on the inhalation and hold each pose for one exhalation.

**Inhale:** Start on hands and knees

**Exhale:** Move to next pose (downward facing dog pose or child's pose)

### 🌿 downward-facing dog pose 🌿

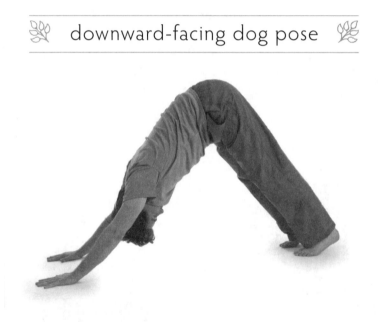

Downward-facing dog releases tension in the legs, hips, chest, and back, while building strength in the upper body.

**Do:** From an all-fours position, lift your knees and begin to lift your hips. Press down through the hands and draw your shoulders and hips back and up. Slowly straighten your legs to increase the stretch, or keep your knees bent if this is more comfortable.

**Feel:** The connection of the hands to the ground and the sensation of strength in the upper body; the connection of the feet to the ground and the sensation of stretch in the lower body; the flow of breath in and out of your nose, mouth, and throat.

## ❧ child's pose ❧

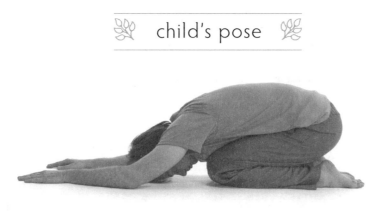

Child's pose releases tension in the hips, back, shoulders, and chest and is a full-body gesture of trust in, and gratitude for, the present moment.

Do: Drop to your knees, draw your hips back toward the heels, rest your belly on your thighs, and rest the arms and head on the ground. If your hips cannot touch your heels, or your knees are uncomfortable as you hold this pose, place a pillow or blanket between the hips and heels.

Feel: The movement of breath in the belly and back, and a sense of gratitude in your mind and heart.

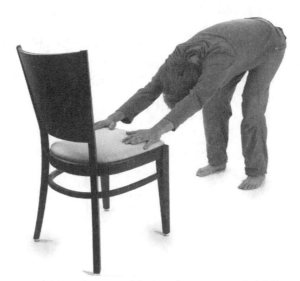

Chair pose combining downward facing-dog pose and child's pose

# COBRA RISING
# (COBRA POSE AND RESTING COBRA)

This sequence powerfully strengthens the back of the body and teaches you how to maintain a balance of effort and ease.

**Start:** Lying on belly

**Inhale:** Cobra pose

**Exhale:** Resting cobra

## cobra pose

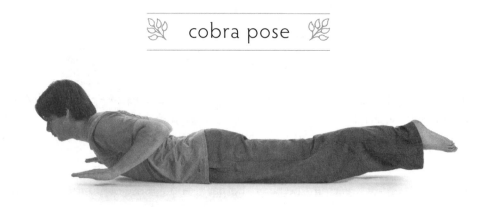

This pose strengthens the back and legs and embodies the ability to rise above adversity.

**Do:** Bring your arms by your side, either bent with your hands by your chest or stretched straight back alongside your hips. As you inhale, lift your head, shoulders, chest, and legs. Come up only as far as you can maintain a comfortable breath. When holding the pose, stay at 50 to 60 percent maximum effort and allow the height of the pose to naturally rise and fall a bit as you breathe.

**Feel:** The strength of your back body, the openness of your chest as you inhale, and the subtle rise and fall of the upper body as you breathe.

## resting cobra

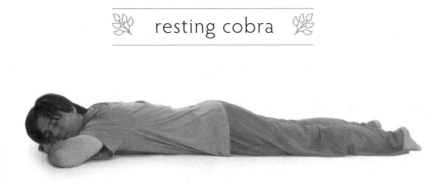

This pose is an opportunity to practice resting and receiving support when effort is no longer needed.

**Do:** Relax on your belly. Make a comfortable resting place for your arms and head.

**Feel:** The support of the ground underneath you and the movement of the breath in your belly and back.

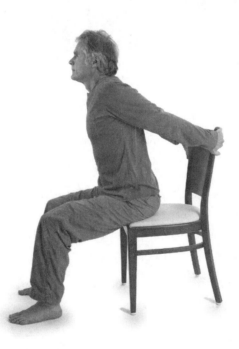

Chair cobra combining benefits of rising and resting cobra

# THE DRAWBRIDGE
## (BRIDGE POSE AND KNEES-TO-CHEST POSE)

The drawbridge strengthens and stretches the entire body.

**Start:** Lying on your back, with legs bent and feet on the ground, knees and feet hips-distance apart

**Inhale:** Bridge pose

**Exhale:** Knees-to-chest pose

## 🌿 bridge pose 🌿

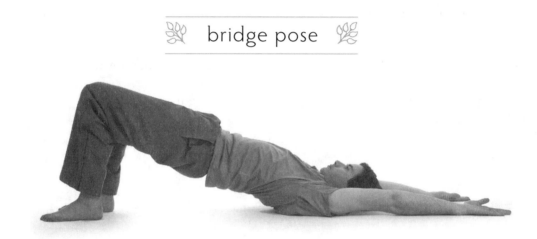

Bridge pose builds strength in the legs, hips, and core and releases tension in the shoulders and chest.

**Do:** In one smooth movement, lift your arms toward the ceiling and then lower them to the floor behind you, as you press down through your heels to lift your hips and lower back off the ground. Keep your knees right over your feet, not falling out to the sides or squeezing together.

**Feel:** The connection of your feet to the ground, the strength of your legs, and the movement of the breath in your belly, rib cage, and chest.

## 🌿 knees-to-chest pose 🌿

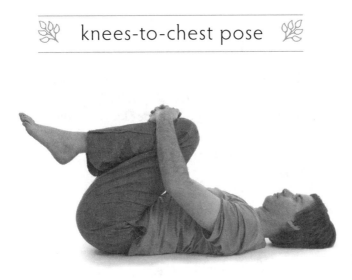

Knees-to-chest pose releases tension in the hips and back.

**Do:** Hug your knees into your belly and chest. Keep your head and shoulders relaxed on the ground.

**Feel:** The support of the ground underneath you and the movement of the belly against your legs as you breathe.

# SWEET DREAMS
## (CRADLE POSE, RESTING TWIST, AND HALF MOON POSE)

This sequence is made of three reclining poses. It is a lullaby for the body and a perfect transition into the final relaxation pose. You can practice each pose on both sides of the body before moving on to the next pose, or practice all three poses on one side of the body before switching sides and starting the sequence over. This sequence works best as a slow flow, holding each pose for at least five to ten breaths before moving to the next pose.

### cradle pose

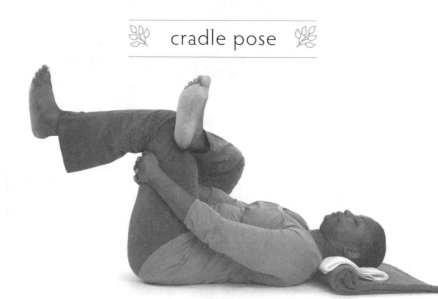

Cradle pose releases tension in the hips, groin, and back.

**Do:** Cross one ankle over the opposite leg, near the knee. Draw the bottom leg in toward your belly and clasp your hands behind the thigh or across the shin. Keep your head and shoulders relaxed on the ground.

**Feel:** The sensation of stretch in your outer hip and inner thigh, the heaviness of your shoulders and head resting on the floor, and the rise and fall of your belly as you breathe.

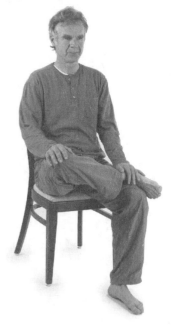

## resting twist

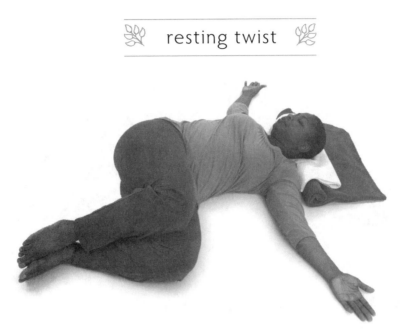

Resting twist releases tension in the belly, chest, shoulders, spine, and hips and naturally deepens the breath.

**Do:** Start with both knees over your belly and then drop both legs to one side. Stretch your arms out to either side. Do not force your legs, shoulders, or arms to the ground if they do not naturally touch. Relax and let gravity draw you into the pose. You can always place a blanket or pillow underneath any part of the body that does not touch the ground.

**Feel:** The sense of gravity bringing you into the pose, the support of the ground underneath you, and the inhalation stretching the belly and chest from the inside out.

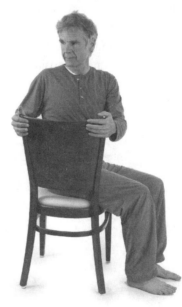

## ❧ half moon pose ❧

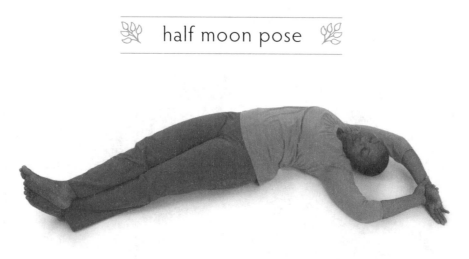

Half moon pose releases tension along the whole side of the body and is an opportunity to practice doing less to receive more.

**Do**: Start lying on your back. Walk both heels to one side until you feel a stretch in the outer thigh or hip. Cross one ankle over the other. Press your elbows down to lift the shoulders and move them over in the same direction as your heels. Rest your arms on the ground overhead and pull them gently into the stretch. Keep feet, hips, shoulders, and arms on the ground.

**Feel**: The sensations of stretch along the side of legs, hips, waist, chest, and shoulders; the connection of your heels, hips, shoulders, head, and hands to the ground; the inhalation stretching the belly and chest from the inside out.

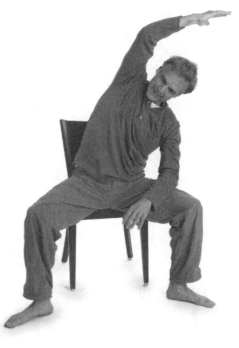

## ❧ relaxation pose ❧

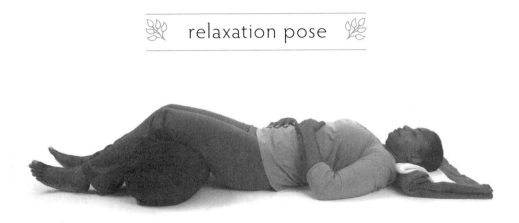

Always finish a movement practice with relaxation. The traditional way to end a yoga movement session is to lie down on your back, in relaxation pose, close your eyes, and rest for five to fifteen minutes. If this is not a comfortable position for you, see chapter 6 for different relaxation poses and strategies.

### The Letting Go Checklist: Places to Check for Unnecessary Tension in Each Pose

Every active yoga pose should be a balance of effort (intentional tension to create strength) and ease (letting go of any tension that doesn't directly support you in a pose). As you hold each pose, scan your body for unnecessary tension. Below is a list of the most common places people habitually hold unnecessary tension in yoga poses and in everyday life. In each pose, check whether you are tensing any of the following areas of your body. If so, can you relax the area while still supporting yourself in the pose? Check:

- jaw/mouth
- forehead/eyes
- neck
- shoulders/upper back

- lower back/middle back
- belly
- hips
- fingers/hands

If you do this kind of body scan regularly in your yoga practice, you will find yourself carrying less unconscious tension in the rest of your life as well.

## putting it together

Once you've explored the poses in this chapter, you're ready to put them together with what you've already learned. Below are some ideas for integrating movement with the practices you've learned for breathing and befriending the body.

- The breath-freeing series of stretches in chapter 3 (p. 30) are a perfect way to begin any movement practice. Use them to prepare the body and center the mind.

- Let Listening to Your Body (p. 61) inspire your movement practice. Practice Hands-on Breath Awareness (p. 26) for a couple of minutes and then ask your body, "What poses/stretches do you need today?" Let you inner wisdom lead you toward a specific set of poses.

- Practice breath awareness in every movement and pose. It will make each movement a healing meditation, and each pose safer and more comfortable.

- To seal in the benefits of a movement practice, practice Breathing the Body (p. 61) as you rest in your final relaxation pose.

- Relaxation pose following a movement session is a wonderful time to practice breathing techniques for pain relief. Because you are relaxed, it will be easier to learn the techniques. Practicing them regularly in a relaxed state will also build your confidence and willingness to use them when you are in pain.

- Have you discovered a pose that challenges your flexibility or strength? These are the poses you might be tempted to skip, rush through, or grit your teeth and suffer through. Instead, can you take the attitude of befriending your body and view these poses as gifts to your body? Instead of pushing your body through them, can you let your body receive them? If you soften your attitude toward these poses, you might be surprised at how much you come to like these poses and the positive change they can create in your body.

# Chapter 6

# relaxation

a student once said to me, "When I hear you say, 'Relax your shoulders,' I agree with you that I need to relax my shoulders. But I don't have any idea *how* to relax my shoulders."

Maybe you can relate. Relaxation sounds like the easiest thing in the world until you try to relax, and all of a sudden it's impossible. You give the command to relax, but the mind and body can be uncooperative in so many ways! From racing thoughts to muscles that refuse to let go, what's supposed to be blissful can become stressful. And when you are in pain, lying down and closing your eyes can be downright frightening, as you find yourself with nothing to do but feel and think about your pain.

If this description of relaxation has you thinking it might be a good idea to skip to the next chapter, hold on. Full relaxation of mind and body is possible and, yes, as blissful as its promise. It is, in fact, the ideal remedy for both chronic stress and pain. This chapter will teach you step-by-step how to relax with two yoga relaxation techniques, conscious relaxation and restorative yoga.

## how relaxation can relieve your pain

Relaxation training has been shown to reduce pain and improve quality of life for people suffering from chronic headaches (D'Souza et al. 2008), back pain (van Tulder, Koes, and Malmivaara 2006), fibromyalgia (Menzies and Kim 2008), osteoarthritis (Morone and Greco 2007), temporomandibular disorders (Riley et al. 2007), and irritable bowel syndrome (Keefer and Blanchard 2002), among many other forms of pain.

Why is relaxation so helpful for chronic pain? To begin with, relaxation is immediately healing. It turns off the stress response and directs the body's energy to growth, repair, immune function, digestion, and other self-nurturing processes. Physician Herbert Benson named this healing mode the "relaxation response" (Benson 1975).

Relaxation also works over the long term to create a clean slate for the mind and body. The relaxation response unravels the mind-body samskaras that contribute to pain and provides the foundation for healing habits. Consistent relaxation practice teaches the mind and body how to rest in a sense of safety rather than chronic emergency. When the body and mind feel safe, it is easier to guide them toward the experience of deep inner joy and peace.

## relaxing during pain

Can you relax even while you are in pain? Yes. It's not only possible, it should become one of your first strategies when you find your pain getting worse. Pain is exactly the time to try a relaxation practice, even if the experience is not as blissful as relaxation when you aren't in pain. As long as the position you are in is not making your pain worse, give relaxation a chance to reveal its benefits to you. Relaxation can work in mysterious ways, including giving you a greater sense of control over your pain and courage to handle your pain.

Relaxation also trains the mind and body to separate the sensations of physical pain from a full-out emergency response. This is why relaxation helps even if it doesn't take away all of your pain. If you can relax even when you are in physical pain, you can untangle the knots in your nervous system that connect all forms of pain and distress. Most people with chronic pain find that pain automatically triggers a stress response, and stress automatically worsens pain. When the knots linking physical pain and stress are untangled, you can break this cycle. The mind and body learn to have more nuanced reactions to life's challenges. If you can learn to relax while in pain, you will find that stress and pain are no longer the mind-body's automatic response to every difficult moment.

# Megan's Story: Finding a Sense of Safety

Megan, a college student double-majoring in economics and philosophy, was struggling to keep up with her classes because of irritable bowel syndrome (IBS). She suffered frequent but unpredictable bouts of abdominal pain and diarrhea. An episode always started with cramps, followed by anxiety about getting sick, and then at least an hour of more severe symptoms. When she was sick, she missed class and couldn't do much of anything until the symptoms passed.

Megan knew that the episodes of IBS were related to stress. She often got sick on the day of an exam, and sometimes even missed exams because she was too sick to leave her dorm. Megan also realized that her panic when she felt the first twinge of abdominal discomfort was making each episode worse—possibly even triggering the full-blown symptom cycle. To top it off, Megan felt a lot of anxiety about the lack of privacy she had. Because she lived in a small dorm room with a roommate and shared the hall bathroom with an entire floor, she had little time alone. So when she was sick, she felt even less in control and more vulnerable to her symptoms.

At the suggestion of a resident advisor in her dorm, Megan found her way into a group yoga class aimed at reducing stress. Her favorite part of class was relaxation. Relaxation created a kind of safe space she could withdraw into, and she always felt better afterward.

Megan started to practice relaxation in her dorm room bed, especially when she felt sick. This strategy turned out to be a true solution for her IBS. When Megan was able to practice relaxation at the first signs of pain, she felt better able to tolerate the discomfort in her abdomen. She imagined the sensations to be tension rather than signs that something was seriously wrong. After she relaxed the rest of her body with conscious relaxation, she imagined her breath dissolving the tension in her abdomen. Megan repeated the phrase "I am safe" as she rested in relaxation pose, which helped relax her mind and prevent her from catastrophizing her symptoms.

Often this process prevented a full-blown attack. As the episodes became shorter and less disruptive, Megan felt less at the mercy of her unpredictable digestive tract. It was then that she realized how much the IBS was contributing to her stress—at least as much as stress had been contributing to the IBS.

If your pain is related to stress, of if you have a tendency to catastrophize pain signals, relaxation can be a wonderful tool for preventing and relieving symptoms. Like Megan, you may find that not every sensation of discomfort inevitably leads to a major episode of pain. Relaxation can become a way to let your mind and body know that you are safe.

# THE PRACTICES

## CONSCIOUS RELAXATION

*Consciously tense and relax the body, one area at a time. Rest between areas.*

*Practice:*

- *Lying down, or in any other position if lying down is not comfortable.*

- *To release stress and tension in the body.*

- *During stress or pain episodes to shift attention and to find a sense of safety, control, and comfort.*

- *In bed before sleep to help overcome insomnia related to pain or stress.*

*A full-body practice will take five to ten minutes.*

Let's try a little experiment in relaxation: lift your shoulders as high as you can to your ears. Squeeze them tight! Now let go, and let the shoulders drop. Do this again, only this time with the breath: inhale as you lift your shoulders as high as you can, and exhale through your mouth as you drop them. Now, do it again, only lift your shoulders half as high, using only half the effort and tension. Do this one more time, with even less effort, lifting the shoulders only a little. Exhale, and let go completely.

The next step requires closing your eyes. You're going to repeat the whole process, but in your imagination only. With your eyes closed, imagine lifting your shoulders as high as you can to your ears as you inhale and dropping them as you exhale. Do this a few times, imagining tension and then imagining relaxation. Imagine full effort, then half effort, then half that effort. Then rest your shoulders and notice your breath. Keep your eyes closed and take a few moments to simply notice how you feel.

So, how did it go? Were you able to tense your shoulders on purpose? If so, you've taken an important first step in learning how to relax. Intentional tension may seem like a step in the wrong direction, but it can actually help reprogram the body and mind for relaxation.

Here's why: most of the tension you hold in your body is unconscious and unintentional. This is one way chronic pain can sneak up on you—unconscious habits of tension fly underneath the radar until suddenly the tension turns into pain. The problem is, you can't let go of tension you aren't aware of and aren't doing on purpose.

The yoga practice of conscious relaxation follows the principle that it is easier to undo something you are doing on purpose than something you are doing unconsciously. During conscious relaxation, you will tense different areas of your body on purpose and then let go of that effort. Just as you did with your shoulders in the relaxation experiment, you will start with big movement and work your way toward more subtle tension and release. The rounds that use only your imagination work at a deeper level of retraining the mind and body. Imagery acts on even unconscious tension, allowing this round to dissolve tension you cannot manipulate at will.

Over time, you will find that a regular practice of conscious relaxation makes it easier to drop into the healing state of the full relaxation response. You will also gain greater awareness of when and where you hold tension in your body. With this awareness and the skill of conscious relaxation, you will be able to let go of that tension at will.

## Getting Started

Conscious relaxation can be practiced in any position that you find comfortable, including seated, standing, or lying down.

Start with an area of your body that you feel like you have more conscious control over. This likely will not be any area of your body where you chronically hold tension or experience pain. Work your way to those chronically tense and painful areas after you have established relaxation in other areas of the body. If you have a history of muscle spasms or injuries in an area, skip the first step of the process (full tension) and start with one of the gentle versions, either using less effort or starting with the imagination round.

## Rotating Conscious Tension and Relaxation Around the Body

Follow the guidelines below for any or all of these areas of your body:

- hands and wrists
- arms
- shoulders and neck
- face
- chest
- belly
- back
- hips
- legs
- feet and ankles

## Creating Tension and Letting Go

There are many ways to tense a body part. Don't worry about whether you are doing it exactly the right way. In the first round, create the kind of tension that moves the part of the body you are working with. Squeeze, lift, tighten, contract, pull, push—whatever makes sense for that body part. To let go, simply stop doing the active tension. The result will by definition be relaxation. Repeat the movement a few times, but with progressively less effort and tension each time.

In the imagination rounds, close your eyes and visualize the actions you just performed. Imagine the feeling of the tension and release. You may find that imagining tensing and letting go continues to release tension, even though you are no longer actively tensing the muscle first. This is natural and a good sign that the process is working. If the imagination round feels confusing or difficult, you can leave it out. You may find it easier, at first, to work with only the big tense-and-release round, as this will be easier to control. In this case, you can add the imagination round in later sessions.

## Breathing

You will notice that sometimes it is easier to create tension when you inhale (for example, the shoulder or back) and sometimes it is easier to create tension when you exhale (for example, the belly or hips). The most important thing is to make the breath a part of this process. Experiment with your breathing to see which areas tense more naturally on the exhalation and which tense more naturally on the inhalation. As long as you are not holding your breath, whatever pattern you follow is just fine. Be sure to rest in a relaxed breath between rounds of tensing and releasing the body.

## Resting

Between body areas, pause for a couple of breaths and notice how you feel. To deepen the effects of conscious relaxation, you can use the visualization of Breathing the Body (p. 45) for each area of the body after you consciously tense and relax it. Imagine inhaling and exhaling from each part of the body, and imagine any lingering tension being dissolved by the breath. You can also use a light/color visualization during the resting phase. After you consciously tense and release an area of the body, close your eyes and imagine that area softly glowing with light or a color you associate with healing, comfort, and relaxation. By the time you are finished with the entire practice, you can imagine the whole body radiant with light or your healing color.

# restorative yoga

Restorative yoga turns on the healing relaxation response by combining gentle yoga poses with conscious breathing and meditation. In the following pages, you will learn five restorative yoga poses that may be practiced on their own or in a sequence.

There are a few things that make restorative yoga so relaxing. First, each pose is meant to be held for longer than a few breaths. You can stay in a restorative pose for ten minutes or even longer. The stillness allows the body to drop even the deepest layers of tension.

Second, restorative poses use props to support your body. Props can include the wall, a chair, a couch, pillows, blankets, towels, or bolsters designed especially for restorative yoga practice. The right support in a pose will make it feel effortless, so your body can fully let go.

You also shouldn't feel strong sensations of stretch or strength the way you might in a more active yoga pose. Stretching and strengthening, although healthy, are both forms of tension in the body. They are a kind of good stress on the body, asking the body to adapt to the challenges of a pose. Restorative yoga is all about letting go of stress and tension. You will adapt the poses to your body, using whatever props make your body feel wonderful exactly as it is. As you hold each pose, look for a quality of ease in the body and the breath that seems light or even neutral.

Finally, although these poses may look as though you are doing nothing, this is far from the truth. Restorative yoga rests the body but engages the mind. The breathing and meditation elements of each pose make restorative yoga an active process of focusing the mind on healing thoughts, sensations, and emotions.

## How to Practice Restorative Yoga: General Guidelines

The following guidelines will help you discover the healing potential of restorative yoga.

### make each pose comfortable

Take your time setting yourself up in a pose so that you will feel comfortable resting in the pose. Pay particular attention to the instructions for choosing and arranging your props.

None of these poses should introduce new discomfort or make existing pain worse. As a comparison, you can use your typical level of comfort while sitting or lying down. If the pose is physically uncomfortable, see if there is a way to adjust the props or your body to make yourself comfortable. If that is not possible, try a different restorative pose. There is nothing magical about being able to practice all of these poses. If you can find relaxation in any one of them, you will receive the benefits of a restorative yoga practice.

Once you are supported in a pose and feel as comfortable as possible, commit to that pose. Be still. Even small adjustments and movements can keep you from falling into a state of deep relaxation. Close your eyes and turn your attention to your breathing.

Rather than set a strict predetermined time for how long to stay in a pose, start with soft guidelines to hold each pose for a couple of minutes. You can extend this length of time as it feels nurturing and helpful, and you should always come out of a pose that is creating new discomfort or pain. If you are concerned about falling asleep in a pose, you can set a timer for ten or fifteen minutes. That way, your mind won't need to monitor time or worry about staying awake.

### remember to breathe

Practice relaxed breathing in restorative poses. A soft, easy breath promotes physical relaxation. Breath awareness is a wonderful way to keep the mind relaxed and free of worries or distractions. As you rest in each pose, notice how it feels to inhale and exhale. Let these sensations be a conscious alternative to stressful thoughts or sensations of pain. If you are practicing a restorative pose to find relief from pain, you may want to practice the Relief Breath (p. 41).

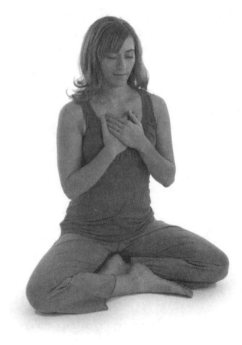

### keep a mental focus

Because there is nothing physical to do in relaxation, you may find that your mind wanders. It is helpful to have a mental focus that reinforces the physical and emotional benefits of a restorative practice. The breath can be a point of focus, but other meditation techniques may be helpful as well.

In the instructions for each pose, you will find one or more suggested meditations. Holding a phrase or image in your mind can make it easier to rest in the stillness of the pose. Experiment with how it feels to focus the mind with a meditation. If it feels distracting or like too much work, simply drop that part of the practice and let the mind rest on the sensations of breathing.

## Selecting Poses and Sequencing

The order of poses presented here is just one possible sequence. As you explore the poses, you may find that your body prefers a different sequence or that you would rather stay longer in one pose than practice several poses for shorter periods. You can also integrate restorative poses into an active yoga session (using the poses in chapter 5). See the sample practices in chapter 8 for ideas about how to include restorative poses in a full yoga practice.

As you try each pose, look for one that feels like home. Which pose feels the most supportive, comforting, and safe? This will become part of your therapeutic yoga practice for difficult times—a pose that you can turn to when you need relief from physical or emotional overwhelm.

## What You Will Need

As in an active yoga practice, wear comfortable clothes that do not interfere with breathing or movement.

A variety of props can be used interchangeably in restorative yoga. In general, it will be helpful to have several pillows and blankets ready before you begin. Other possible props include a couch, chair, wall, towels, an eye pillow, yoga blocks, and bolsters designed especially for restorative yoga practice. Use whatever you have handy, and improvise as needed. If you'd like to invest in tools specifically designed to support yoga practice, see the resources section at the end of the book.

You may want to have an easy-to-set timer to keep track of time (and wake you up if you fall asleep). Relaxing music can also be a wonderful complement to a restorative yoga practice.

## ❧ supported inversion ❧

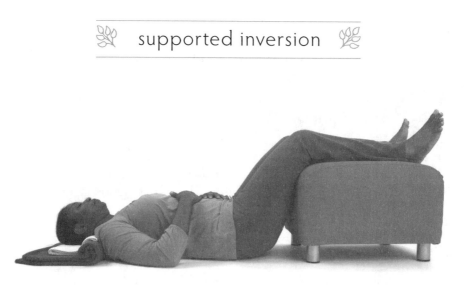

## Benefits

This pose relaxes the back and hips without overstretching them. Poses that gently bring the legs above the heart also improve circulation and have a calming effect on many systems of the body, including the nervous system and cardiovascular system.

## Props

A wall, chair, or sofa. Optional: a small rolled towel or blanket to support your neck and head, and an eye pillow or a cloth to drape over your eyes.

## Instructions

Seat yourself on the floor near the wall or your chair, with one side of your body facing the wall or chair. If you are using extra support for your head and neck, place it where your head will rest, about one arm's length away from the wall or chair. Start to lean back on your arms and let your hips turn as you raise your legs onto the support of the wall or chair, until you find yourself lying comfortably on your back. Have your legs stretched upward and resting on the wall or bent on the chair. If you are at the wall, make sure that you do not feel a strain behind the knees, in the back of your legs and hips, or in your lower back. If you do, try the pose with hips further away from the wall, to reduce pressure on the legs and back. If you continue to feel any strain in the wall version, you may find the bent-leg version using a chair or sofa much more comfortable. Let yourself relax into the support of the pose.

## Breathing

Once you are settled in the pose, bring your hands to rest on your belly. Feel the belly rise and fall as you breathe. Supported inversion is also a perfect pose for practicing the Balancing Breath visualization (p. 43).

## Meditation

This pose is in invitation to drop your usual worries and burdens. As you inhale, say silently in your mind, "Let," and as you exhale, "go."

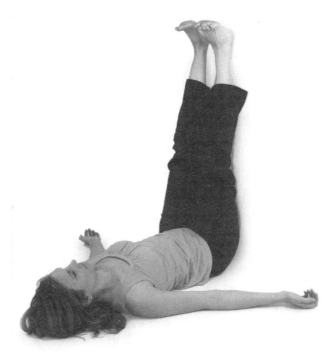

## ❧ nesting pose ❧

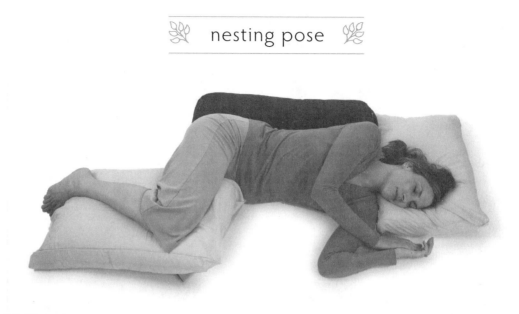

## Benefits

Nesting pose creates a sense of security and nurturing. It may also be a position you are comfortable sleeping in, making it an excellent posture to practice if you have insomnia or other difficulty sleeping.

## Props

Two to three pillows. Optional: a yoga bolster.

## Instructions

Lie on your side, legs bent and drawn in toward your belly. Rest your head on a pillow, and place a pillow or bolster between your knees. Rest your arms in whatever position feels most comfortable. If available, another bolster or pillow may be placed behind your back for an extra sense of support. For a balancing counterpose, nesting pose can be followed with a resting twist (holding for ten breaths), as shown on the next page.

## Breathing

Rest in the natural rhythm of your breath, observing each inhalation and exhalation as it moves through the body. Take comfort in the simplicity and effortlessness of this action.

## Meditation

Nesting pose is about feeling safe and supported, both in your body and in all areas of your life. Repeat silently in your mind, "I am safe" or "I am supported." If there are other words, images, or memories that make you feel safe and supported, bring them to mind.

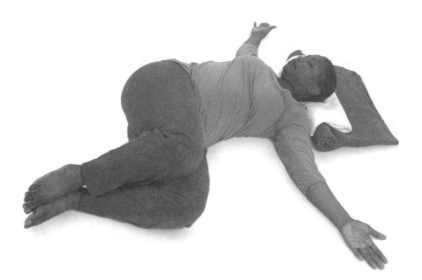

## 🌿 supported bound angle pose 🌿

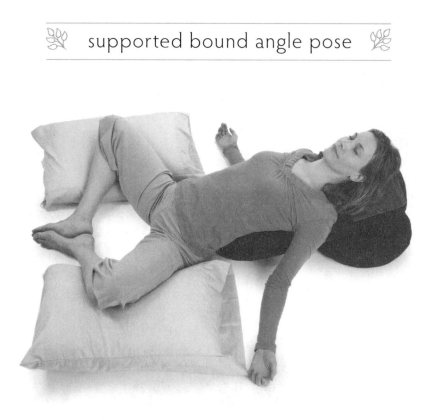

## Benefits

This pose relaxes tension in the belly, chest, and shoulders. The pose can inspire a feeling of abundance, providing an opportunity to reflect on all you are grateful for.

## Props

Two pillows or small blankets and one bolster or very sturdy cushion. You will also need something to rest one end of the bolster on. Almost anything can be used for the end support, including a yoga block or stack of telephone books. Optional: an eye pillow or small towel or cloth.

## Instructions

Lean the bolster on a block or other support. Sit in front of the bolster with your legs in a diamond shape. Place a pillow or rolled blanket under each knee, making sure that the legs are fully supported without a deep stretch or strain in the knees, legs, or hips. Lean back onto the bolster so that you are supported from the lower back to the back of the head. Rest your arms wherever is most comfortable.

## Breathing

This pose relaxes tension in the belly and chest that otherwise can restrict the breath. Notice the whole front of your body relax and gently stretch open as you inhale. Follow this sensation and feel the ease in the front of the body as you breathe.

## Meditation

Bring to mind specific things you are grateful for, imagining each one in detail until you feel an authentic sense of gratitude. Imagine saying to each one, "Thank you."

## 🌿 supported backbend pose 🌿

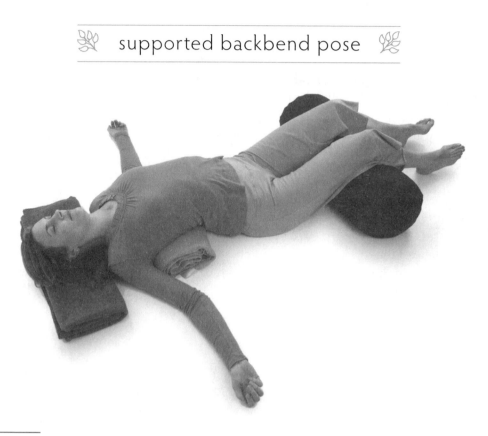

## Benefits

Supported backbend is a heart-opening pose that reinforces your desire to embrace life and not let challenges—including pain—separate you from life. This pose also works magic to release chronic tension in the back and shoulders, undoing postural habits that come from spending too much time at a desk, at a computer, or driving.

## Props

One or more folded pillows or rolled blanket/towels to support the upper body. A bolster or stack of pillows or blankets to support the lower body. A rolled towel or small blanket to support your head and neck.

## Instructions

Sitting, place a bolster or stack of pillows or blankets under slightly bent knees. Place one folded pillow or rolled blanket/towel behind you; when you lie back, it should support the upper rib cage, not the lower back. If you need extra support underneath the lower rib cage and lower back, roll a small towel to support the natural curve of the spine.

Place a rolled towel or small blanket to support your head and neck at whatever height is most comfortable.

## Breathing

This pose improves the flow of the breath in the upper chest, rib cage, and belly. Allow yourself to feel this movement as you inhale and exhale. Imagine breathing in and out through your heart center. Visualize the movement of breath from your heart to your lungs as you inhale and from the lungs back out through the heart center as you exhale.

## Meditation

Imagine the sun, radiant and nourishing, in your heart center. Feel the subtle expansion and contraction of your chest as you breathe, and imagine the sun radiating in unison with the breath. Repeat silently in your mind, "My heart is open."

# ✿ supported forward bend ✿

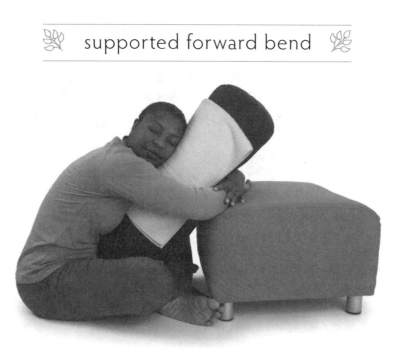

## Benefits

Supported forward bend relaxes the hips and back, unraveling the stress of daily activities on the spine. Hugging the bolster and resting your head on its support provides a natural sense of security and comfort.

## Props

A chair, sofa, or stack of pillows/blankets to lean on. Optional: a yoga bolster to hug and rest your head on.

## Instructions

Sit cross-legged on the floor. Lean forward onto the support of a sofa, chair, or stack of pillows, blankets, or cushions. If you have a bolster, place one end in your lap and the other end on the sofa, chair, or stack of support. Rest your head on whatever support is available. If you are using the bolster, you can hug it in any way that feels comfortable, turning your head to the side. Be sure that whatever support you are using is high enough and sturdy enough to support you, without creating strain in the back or hips. If you feel a strong stretch that is uncomfortable to hold, you need more support.

## Breathing

In this pose, the belly, chest, and back all expand and contract with each breath. Feel the movement of the whole torso as you inhale and exhale. Feel your belly and chest gently press into the support of the bolster/pillows as you inhale. Let the sensation of your breath deepen the sensation of being hugged.

## Meditation

Imagine some place where you would feel completely at peace. For many people, this might be a place in nature, a place of worship, or the idea of being surrounded by loved ones. Imagine yourself in this setting, bringing to mind any sensations—sights, sounds, smells, or touch—that help you connect to the experience of peace.

If you are practicing this pose for relief from pain or suffering, consider repeating a phrase in your mind that you find personally comforting, such as "This too shall pass" or "God loves me."

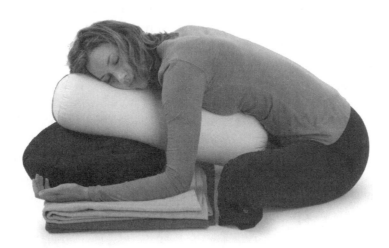

## Lisa's Story: Finding Hope

Lisa's fatigue was both mysterious and maddening. When it first showed up during the winter holidays, she thought it was just the flu combined with exhaustion from overdoing things. But as the holidays passed and her fatigue didn't, her family became alarmed and encouraged her to see a doctor. Her general physician couldn't give her a definite diagnosis and referred her to a specialist. The specialist gave her lots of tests but also couldn't tell Lisa for sure what was causing her exhaustion. Eventually Lisa was diagnosed with chronic fatigue syndrome. By this time, she had taken an extended sick leave from work and was wondering if she would ever be able to return.

Lisa's physician gave her two prescriptions: an anti-inflammatory drug and an antidepressant. What she wasn't given was an explanation for why she was so tired or any answers about when or even whether she would recover.

To Lisa, the lack of medical understanding meant lack of hope. Her growing sense of hopelessness was accompanied by greater fatigue. Some days she was so tired, she crawled back into bed less than an hour after waking. The worst part was that even though she was almost always exhausted, she had trouble sleeping. This left her plenty of time alone with her worries and frustrations. She described it as a "wide-awake nightmare."

Without a clear path for recovery, Lisa needed some way to feel like she was taking care of herself. She wanted to be able to do something every day that felt like an active step toward improving her energy and mood. Lisa didn't have the strength for exercise, but she found great solace in restorative yoga. It was something she could do every day, knowing that it made her feel better both physically and emotionally.

Lisa kept her yoga mat and props out so that there would be no barrier to practicing. She took great care in choosing inspirational music to play while she practiced, knowing that her favorite songs would lift her spirits. She took seriously the idea that focusing on gratitude, joy, connection, and courage could change the state of her body. She chose one meditation each day to practice in her final restorative pose, imagining the thoughts and sensations of each meditation restoring her strength and well-being.

Lisa thought of her restorative yoga practice as her third daily prescription. It became the one part of her self-care program that consistently made her feel optimistic about her future.

Many types of pain and illness are physically and emotionally overwhelming, especially when they pull you out of your normal life and put you into the role of patient. When pain or illness is this overwhelming, even a few minutes of focusing on health can restore hope and inspire courage in the journey of healing. Whenever you find yourself lowest in spirit, you can always turn to yoga to affirm the part of you that is healthy and whole, despite pain or illness.

## putting it together

Relaxation is a wonderful stand-alone practice, but it can also be used to enhance the healing benefits of other yoga practices:

- Use a favorite restorative yoga pose as the foundation for any breathing or befriending-the-body practice (see chapters 3 and 4).

- Relaxation is usually practiced at the end of an active yoga session. However, you can practice full-body conscious relaxation at the beginning of a session to release unconscious tension that would otherwise make the active poses less comfortable.

- For days when you have less energy or simply want a gentle practice for the body, combine the Freeing the Breath series (p. 30) with restorative yoga poses.

# Chapter 7

# meditation

In chapter 4, you learned how to befriend your body, and in chapter 5, you learned how to move your body. Meditation is yoga's way of befriending and moving the mind.

The meditations you will learn in this chapter will show you how to make your own mind a safe place to be. You will also learn how to move the mind away from stress, pain, and suffering and guide it toward wisdom and joy.

## how meditation relieves chronic pain

Yogis have long used meditation to alter pain and stress, but only recently has research looked at how meditation works.

## Changing the Mind and Body

Stress and pain focus your attention on what is wrong. Continued attention to these sensations, thoughts, and emotions keeps you in a state of suffering. Meditation can interrupt a stress or pain response by shifting your attention. Studies show that focusing on the breath, a mantra, or a visualization can quickly move the mind and body from a state of stress to a state of relaxation (Bernardi et al. 2001; Wu and Lo 2008) and also increase tolerance for pain (Grant and Rainville 2009).

In one unusual study, researchers in Japan tested a master yogi who claimed to be able to block all pain during meditation (Kakigi et al. 2005). The researchers used a laser to create a pain response in the yogi, both before and during meditation. Brain imaging revealed normal pain processing when the yogi was not meditating. During meditation, however, there was dramatically reduced activity in all the brain areas associated with a pain response, including the areas that produce pain sensations, thoughts and emotions about pain, and the stress response. Although most of us will never become master yogis, this study demonstrates the full potential of meditation for changing your experience of pain.

Meditation does not just interrupt negative states of mind; it also produces positive states of mind. While all meditation techniques can be healing, the focus of the meditation determines which specific changes take place. For example, research shows that a meditation on joy activates the areas of the brain that produce positive emotions, a meditation on the body activates areas of the brain associated with sensation and movement, and a meditation using visualization activates areas of the brain associated with whatever is being imagined (Cahn and Polich 2006). These studies confirm what you will experience as you try a variety of meditation techniques: by choosing your focus, you can create a specific state of mind that is both real and healing.

## Transforming Habits of Mind

Meditation does more than temporarily interrupt negative states and replace them with positive states. Many studies show that regular meditation practice can lead to positive long-term changes in pain, mood, stress, and physical health (Bormann et al. 2005; Fredrickson et al. 2008; Lane, Seskevich, and Pieper 2007; Teixeira 2008).

One of the most important ways that meditation creates lasting changes is by helping you discover the habits of your mind that contribute to pain, stress, and suffering. Everyone has chronic, unconscious habits of thinking and feeling. Some patterns, such as chronic worrying, self-criticism, anger, or loneliness, intensify and reinforce chronic pain. Other patterns, such as acceptance, gratitude, or humor, can help reduce or prevent pain.

Your own habits might include worrying about something in the future or reminiscing about a favorite experience. Perhaps you have a habit of criticizing and blaming yourself or a habit of looking for the good in yourself and others. These habits of mind—whether harmful or healing— are strengthened every time you repeat the pattern. With each round of "practice," the mind and body become shaped more and more in the direction of responding to future experiences with the same thoughts and emotions.

It is often easy to see the habits of other people and recognize them as a lens through which they view life. But it is very difficult for us to see ourselves when our thoughts and feelings reflect a habit and not necessarily reality. When they are your own habits, they tend to feel like the only reasonable response to life. This is what makes them so powerful.

Meditation reveals the freedom you have to choose one thought over another. It puts your inner wisdom and joy, rather than the unconscious habits of your mind, in charge of your life experience. Through meditation, you learn to recognize unconscious habits of mind and consciously choose new habits. As you practice the meditation techniques in this chapter, you will discover that you can become a guide for you mind. Rather than letting the mind's habits pull you from one worry or complaint to another, you can move the mind toward specific sensations, thoughts, and emotions. As you do so, you will be transforming old habits that reinforce chronic pain into new habits that support healing.

# the practices you will learn

In this chapter, you will learn four types of meditation: *shamatha* ("befriending the mind"), *mantra* ("protecting the mind"), *citta bhavana* ("moving the mind"), and *pratipaksha bhavana* ("moving the mind in the opposite direction"). All these techniques have two things in common. First, they are rooted in the healing wisdom of yoga philosophy. Second, they have been demonstrated through research or clinical programs to help people with chronic physical or emotional pain.

Shamatha meditation is the practice of resting your mind on the breath and gently guiding it away from thoughts that lead to suffering. You already learned the basis of this meditation, breath awareness, in chapter 3. To practice breath awareness as a meditation, you will simply add awareness of how your mind wanders. Each time the mind wanders, you bring it back to the breath as an act of friendliness, or compassion, toward your mind.

A mantra is a sound, word, or phrase that you repeat either silently in your mind or out loud. The word *mantra* can be translated as the protection ("tra") of the mind ("man"). A mantra can come to your rescue when you are in pain and build a resilience of the mind to protect you from future suffering.

*Citta bhavana* can be translated as consciously creating or choosing ("bhavana") your state of mind ("citta"). These are the meditations that help you choose to experience healing states of mind, such as joy and gratitude. In these practices, you will learn how to focus your attention on healing thoughts and re-create healing sensations and emotions at will.

The final meditation technique, pratipaksha bhavana, is an advanced version of citta bhavana. *Pratipaksha bhavana* literally means "moving the mind in the opposite direction." It is the practice of choosing to change your state of mind when you are feeling stuck in negative thoughts and emotions.

## the meditation myth

Many students have said to me, "I can't meditate. I've tried, but I can't get rid of all my thoughts." They try to empty their minds, only to notice the constant whirl of thoughts and feelings. This feels like failure—and so they give up, convinced that meditation is not for them, or worse, that meditation doesn't work.

If you've had a similar experience, don't worry, and don't give up on meditation yet. Meditation is not about having no thoughts, and it's not about "emptying" the mind. Meditation is about awareness and choice, not mind control. You are becoming a caregiver for your mind. You cannot fail at the meditations described in this chapter, even if you find them challenging at first. To get the most out of them, all you need to do is pay attention to your mind and have the heartfelt intention to move your mind toward healing states.

## getting started

I recommend reading through this entire chapter before choosing a meditation technique to get started with. One will probably seem more appealing to you than the others, and you can trust this intuition. Rather than trying every meditation technique, pick one that you'd like to explore a little bit every day for at least one week. This is the best way to get to know your own mind and to discover the benefits of a meditation technique. Over time, you can explore all of the techniques in this chapter. But if you find one that brings you peace of mind, it is not necessary to add anything else.

You can make meditation a formal practice, such as the first thing you do when you wake up or the last thing you do before you go to sleep. It can also be something you do when you remember, pausing to meditate for a couple of minutes at work or at home. The best way to meditate is whatever way actually gets you to meditate. Forget ideals of sitting for long periods or meditating for a certain amount of time every day. Commit to being a person who meditates and look for opportunities to make it happen.

# THE PRACTICES

## SHAMATHA (BEFRIENDING THE MIND)

*Focus the mind on your breath. Notice each inhalation and each exhalation. Each time the mind wanders to other thoughts, bring it gently back to the breath.*

*Practice:*

- *Seated, if possible, or in any position that is comfortable.*

- *Anytime to befriend the mind and develop greater awareness of how your mind works.*

- *For as little as one minute or as long as desired.*

Befriending the mind (sometimes referred to as *mindfulness meditation*) is the most widely practiced meditation technique. It is also the easiest form of meditation to get started with. The instructions are simple: sit in a comfortable, upright position, close your eyes or face a blank wall, and focus on your breath. Notice each inhalation and each exhalation. Each time your mind wanders from the breath, notice yourself thinking and bring the mind back to the breath.

This meditation is not about paying perfect attention to your breath. Your mind will wander. That's a given. It will wander even when you become quite experienced with this meditation. You may find yourself planning your day, recalling something that happened yesterday, having an imaginary conversation with someone, or even evaluating how well you are meditating (hint: this is one of those habits of mind that leads to suffering, and not part of the meditation instructions!).

Your job is to notice when this happens. The potential for peace of mind is in noticing how the mind wanders and not in achieving some impossible standard of total concentration. Befriending the mind is the practice of becoming aware of samskaras. By sitting still and focusing on the breath, you eliminate external triggers for your mind. The thoughts that show up on the blank screen you've created are the habits of your mind. When the mind has nothing outside itself to grasp onto, it presses "play" on its automatic thoughts and entertains you with stories, memories, fantasies, and worries that have nothing to do with what is actually happening in this moment.

Each time you notice your mind wandering, you have the opportunity to recognize that your thoughts are not the be-all, end-all, final word on reality. This is particularly good news when your thoughts are causing you unnecessary stress and suffering. You do not need to follow the stories just because they came to mind. You can choose not to let yourself get emotionally worked up by each memory, fantasy, or worry. You can choose to refocus on the breath.

Each time you guide yourself back to the breath, it is not because you failed at the meditation but rather because you know that it is the compassionate thing to do for your mind. When you rest the mind on the breath, you experience the peace of mind that comes from consciously letting go of your samskaras. This meditation will teach you how to rest in your own mind, knowing that it is a safe place to be. You have the inner wisdom to recognize when the mind is creating its own suffering, and you have the self-compassion to bring your mind back to the breath.

## How to Practice

When you are ready to try this meditation, you can do it in as little as one minute. Take a comfortable seat, close your eyes, and begin to notice your breath. Notice how it feels to inhale and exhale. You might repeat in your own mind, "Inhale, exhale," if this is helpful. Then, as soon as you notice yourself thinking, congratulate yourself—you have taken the first step to befriending your mind. Then bring your awareness back to your breath. Continue in this way, feeling a sense of delight and not discouragement each time you notice the mind wandering. Softly let the thought go, as if you were releasing a held breath or relaxing a clenched muscle. As you bring your awareness back to the breath, feel a sense of compassion for yourself. If any thought seems particularly difficult to let go, notice this too and simply wish for yourself, "May I be free of this."

You can continue this practice for as long as you like, setting a timer if you are worried about falling asleep.

## Diane's Story: When Thoughts Hurt

Diane loved theater more than anything else in life. At twenty-four years old and just out of college, she was working part time as a costume designer, part time as a drama teacher, and part time as a manager for a local theater company. Her life, though busy, was a dream come true.

The dream was temporarily interrupted by a car accident that left Diane with multiple bone fractures and other injuries. Everyone assured her that she'd be fine in a couple of months. But even after the fractures healed, Diane still had daily pain and stiffness. She felt unable to stop taking her pain medications and worried that her doctors had missed something.

It was hard to get her life back on track, even after the doctors told her she should be able to return to work. Before the accident, it had been easy and even fun to rush from one job to the next and stay up late finishing a project. But now she felt slowed down and held back, a slave to what she thought of as her "broken" body. She frequently found herself thinking, "This pain ruins everything." Diane was angry almost all the time, snapping at friends and coworkers over things that previously would not have bothered her. She justified her anger by telling herself, "Nobody understands my pain."

Diane was still bitter about the accident. She was convinced it was the fault of the other driver and resented the fact that it had been considered an equal-fault accident by the insurance companies. She had revenge fantasies, which she was both obsessed with and ashamed of. Sometimes she replayed the night of the accident, imagining how it might have turned out differently. In some of these alternate-reality versions, she avoided the accident completely; in others, she wasn't lucky enough to survive. None of these scenarios made her feel any better about her current state—they just reminded her of how unpredictable and dangerous life was.

Diane's experience is a classic example of how the mind can be a very unfriendly place. Diane's thoughts about the accident and how it had changed her life created at least as much suffering as the physical pain. This is not unusual; all of Diane's thoughts and emotions are common responses to pain. As common as they are, though, they only lead to misery. The more Diane let her mind follow these thoughts, the more deeply entrenched the patterns became. But because Diane was convinced her thoughts were true, she was unlikely to recognize the choice she had available not to follow them.

In meditation, you learn to be more aware of what's going on in your mind. You can use this awareness to notice how you talk to yourself about pain in everyday life. How often do thoughts like "this pain will never get better" float through your mind? Do you find yourself paying more attention to the things you cannot do or to the evidence that you are coping well? Do you tell yourself "nobody understands my pain," or do you find yourself appreciating the support of your family and friends? Do you imagine the worst outcomes and explanations for every sensation? Or do you reassure yourself that not every pain sensation means something is wrong or getting worse?

How you think about your pain can make a real difference to your pain and functioning. For example, worrying about your pain and expecting the worst can sensitize you to pain by activating the areas of your brain responsible for the sensation, suffering, and stress components of the protective pain response (Gracely et al. 2004). This kind of thinking becomes a self-fulfilling prophecy, with people who catastrophize ending up in worse shape psychologically and finding that pain interferes more with their lives (Hanley et al. 2008). These effects are reversible, however. Using meditation to change the way you think about your pain can reduce pain and improve functioning (Morone et al. 2008).

As you practice noticing your thoughts, you will realize that some thoughts consistently make you suffer. You have the freedom to follow some thoughts and let others go. When you catch yourself in a train of thought that increases your suffering, remember the act of self-compassion you learned in the shamatha meditation: drop the thought and focus your attention on the breath. You can do this anytime—you don't need to be sitting in meditation to be a compassionate guide for your mind. If you practice meditation regularly, you will be less at the mercy of your thoughts and more in control of your life.

# MANTRA MEDITATION

*Repeat a healing sound, word, or phrase silently in your mind or out loud.*

*Practice:*

- *In any position, with eyes open or closed.*

- *Anytime to focus the mind and let go of negative thoughts or emotions.*

- *During stress or pain episodes to shift attention and to find a sense of safety, control, and comfort.*

- *During everyday activities to remind yourself of a healing thought or emotion.*

- *In bed before sleep to help overcome insomnia related to pain or stress.*

- *For as little as one minute or as long as desired.*

A mantra is a healing sound, word, or phrase that you repeat either out loud or silently in your mind. Mantras focus and calm the mind, making mantra meditation a great on-the-spot therapy for anxiety, stress, and insomnia. But mantra meditation is more than a quick fix. Yogis believe that repeating a mantra leaves lasting impressions on the mind. Each time you repeat the mantra, you are reminding yourself of an essential healing truth. With repetition, you will begin to realize and absorb that truth at a deep level.

Mantras can be found in many spiritual traditions, and they can be taken from any inspirational source, including religious texts, songs, or poetry. Prayers are often used as mantras, repeated for spiritual comfort, connection, and healing. The best-known yoga mantra is "om." Like many yoga mantras, *om* has no single meaning but is considered to be an intrinsically sacred and healing sound. In your own practice, you can use the traditional yoga mantras listed below or create your own from any source that inspires you.

## How to Practice

The easiest way to practice mantra meditation is to find a comfortable position with your body, close your eyes, and begin to silently repeat the mantra in your mind. You can do this for as little or as long as you want.

The simple act of repeating a sound or phrase is naturally soothing. But the greatest healing will come when you allow yourself to feel the meaning of the mantra as you repeat it. As you do so, it will be natural to move from a focused mental repetition of the mantra to simply feeling the meaning of the mantra. When this happens, you can let go of repeating the sounds or words and relax with the feeling the mantra evokes.

Saying or singing a mantra out loud has a very different feel to it. Voicing the mantra allows the sound to resonate in your body. It also turns the meditation into a powerful breathing practice. If you choose to experiment with sound, do not worry about pitch or even perfect pronunciation. Let the sound be loud or quiet, as feels right to you.

Once you have found a mantra that inspires you, you can use it during other activities. Mantras can turn any form of exercise, from yoga to walking, into a moving meditation. Even everyday tasks, such as washing the dishes or putting away the laundry, can be done with mantra meditation.

Another way to incorporate mantra into your life is to listen to audio recordings of mantras being chanted or sung (for music labels that produce beautiful and moving mantra recordings, see the resources section at the end of this book). You can listen to a recording as a meditation while resting in a yoga pose or while going about your everyday activities.

## Yoga Mantras to Inspire Peace of Mind and Healing

The sounds of the following traditional mantras are thought to both represent and naturally inspire healing states of mind. Because the sounds themselves are healing, a pronunciation guide is included for each mantra. Focusing on the meaning of the mantra can be equally healing. To help you connect to the meaning, a description and English variation of each mantra is also listed. You can practice mantra meditation with either the traditional sounds or the English variations.

*Om* ("oh-mmm"). This mantra represents the connectedness of all things and the natural goodness or divine that is present in all things. Note that the "mmm" indicates that some time and emphasis should be given to the closing sound of the syllable "m" rather than only extending and emphasizing the vowel sound "oh." The mantra may be repeated out loud or internally. Meditate on the feeling of connection. English variation: "Amen."

*Sat nam* ("saht nahm" or "sah-tah nah-mah"). This mantra represents one's true nature of wisdom and joy. Note that the sound indicated by "ah" refers to the soft "a" sound of "father," which resonates in the throat. The mantra may be repeated out loud or internally. Meditate on the feeling of everything being all right, exactly as it is, and the feeling of being already healthy and already whole, exactly as you are. English variations: "I am already healed and already whole." "Health [joy, wisdom] is my true nature."

*So hum* ("so huh-mmm"). This mantra represents the sound of the breath. Unlike most mantras, it is meant to be repeated only internally, not out loud. As you inhale, mentally think or hear "so"; as you exhale, think or hear "hum." Meditate on the flow of your breath and your connection to life energy. English variation: "Inhale, exhale."

*Om shanti om* ("oh-mmm shahn-tee oh-mmm"). This mantra represents both the direct experience of peace and the desire to share peace with others. May be repeated out loud or internally. Meditate on the feeling of inner peace and acceptance or the desire to forgive or find peace with others. English variation: "As I inhale, I choose peace. As I exhale, I let go."

*Om mani padme hum* ("oh-mmm mah-nee pahd-may huh-mmm"). This mantra represents compassion, connection, and freedom from suffering. May be repeated out loud or internally. Meditate on the feeling of compassion for yourself and others. English variations: "My heart is open. May I be free of this [suffering]."

## Creating Your Own Mantras

Mantras can be any phrase that makes you feel safe, loved, strong, courageous, happy, or at peace. Do you have a favorite prayer, poem, or inspirational saying? Another way to develop your own mantra is to ask yourself, "What do I need to hear?" Is there something you know to be true but nevertheless need permission to remind yourself of? What would relieve your suffering if you really knew in your heart and mind that it was true? How could you express that idea in a phrase or sentence?

Take a few moments to write down some ideas for mantras that you can try in a meditation practice.

# CITTA BHAVANA (MOVING THE MIND)

*Bring to mind the thoughts, sensations, and emotions of a specific healing state.*

*Practice:*

- *In any position with eyes open or closed.*

- *Anytime you want to experience the specific state of mind.*

- *When you first wake up, to set the intention for the day, or right before you go to sleep, as a personal ritual to end the day.*

- *As part of a yoga breathing, movement, or relaxation practice—citta bhavana meditations are excellent additions to most other yoga practices.*

- *For a few minutes every day. Citta bhavana meditations are most healing when they are practiced on a daily basis.*

The following meditations use memories and imagination to create a particular state of mind, such as gratitude and joy.

Many people find it hard to believe that choosing to feel an emotion can have the same effect on your mind and body as it does when the emotion spontaneously happens. But emotions you choose to feel are just as real as the emotions triggered by external events. The changes in your brain and body are the same, and the effects on your mood can be equally powerful. This is both bad and good news.

The bad news is that these emotions are just as real for stress, anger, anxiety, and other unpleasant states of mind. You have probably already noticed that just thinking about something stressful can trigger the same responses in your body—and make you feel just as miserable—as if it were actually happening to you. People don't tend to question how real this self-generated misery is. We all have experience with it, and we know it is real.

The good news is that positive emotions, like gratitude, are healing states whether outside events trigger them or you choose to experience them. For example, choosing to reflect each night on things you are grateful for can lead to very real positive changes in mood and physical health (Emmons and McCullough 2003). Research also shows that when you develop your ability to experience positive states in meditation, you also strengthen your capacity to experience them spontaneously in response to life (Fredrickson et al. 2008).

The more you practice choosing a positive state of mind with citta bhavana meditations, the more you will realize what an empowering and healing technique it can be. Included below are meditations for cultivating gratitude, joy, courage, and connection.

## Meditations for Choosing Gratitude and Joy

Of all the positive emotions you can feel—excitement, hope, pride, fun, love, and so on—gratitude is the easiest to choose. It doesn't require anything in your life to change, and everyone has something to be grateful for. Whenever you want to tap into the experience of deep inner joy, begin with the act of choosing gratitude. The following meditations will help you focus the mind on gratitude and the feelings of joy:

Bring to mind the things in your life that you are grateful for. Allow yourself to feel a sense of gratitude for each. You can practice this as a meditation or a written reflection, adding to your gratitude list each day.

At the end of the day, bring to mind some favorite moments, including moments of pleasure, beauty, humor, connection with others, learning something new, or the satisfaction of being of service and doing good work. As each moment comes to mind, mentally say "thank you."

Bring to mind the memory of a time when someone thanked you. As you think about this time, remember how it felt to be appreciated. See if you can reexperience this feeling now by staying with the memory. Then bring to mind people in your life you could thank. Imagine thanking each person, and imagine how they would feel to be appreciated. Notice how it feels to both extend and receive gratitude.

Bring to mind the memory of a time you felt great joy or deep peace. As you think about this time, recall it in detail and remember how it felt in your body. See if you can reexperience this feeling now. Then see if you can drop the details of the memory and yet stay with the experience of joy and peace in your body in this moment.

Bring to mind the memory of a time when you laughed, or simply imagine laughing about anything. Remember how laughter feels in your body, and see if you can reexperience this feeling now. You may find yourself smiling or even laughing!

After practicing any of these meditations, bring awareness to your breath and body. See if you can stay with how gratitude and joys feels in your body. Realize that these sensations come from your own mind and your own open heart. Gratitude and joy happen inside of you, not to you. To end the meditation, remind yourself, "Joy is my true nature."

# Meditations for Choosing Connection and Courage

You might not associate courage with the sense of being connected to others. Our culture tends to equate courage with risk-taking and a willingness to stand up for yourself. That's all fine and good, but the courage most of us need is the feeling that we can handle whatever happens to us. This kind of courage is rooted not so much in the willingness to jump out of airplanes or to fight for what you want but in a sense of connection to others. It is easier to face life with courage when you know that you are doing it for, or with, others. Fear, on the other hand, is usually rooted in a sense of isolation, loneliness, and the feeling that you are the only person going through whatever you are facing.

There are many meditations on connection that will naturally strengthen your courage for facing everyday challenges, pain, illness, or heartache:

Bring to mind the memory of a time you felt connected to another person, an animal, or nature. A time when you felt affection, love, gratitude, closeness, or being a part of something bigger. As you think about this time, remember how it felt in your body, and see if you can reexperience this feeling now.

At the end of your day, take a moment to review the many people you interacted with that day. Let your mind rest on any person whom you feel a natural sense of connection to or would like to strengthen your sense of connection to. For each person, say in your mind, "Just like me, this person wishes to be healthy. Just like me, this person wishes to be happy. Just like me, this person wishes to be free of suffering. Just like me, this person wishes to know peace." As you allow yourself to feel a sense of connection to each person, add a wish of friendliness: "May you be healthy. May you be happy. May you be free of suffering. May you know peace." This meditation can be a powerful way to forgive others, build friendships, and make you feel more connected to your community.

To choose courage, bring to mind the people who matter most to you in your life or the people who will benefit from you facing what you fear. Allow yourself to feel, in your body, your connection to each person. Allow yourself to feel affection, gratitude, compassion, or a sense of responsibility. Then dedicate your actions to them and feel the natural sense of courage that comes from this commitment.

Dedicate your daily efforts to someone who is suffering and in need of encouragement, support, or healing. Bring this person to mind and feel a sense of compassion for and good will toward this person. Repeat in your mind, "May my actions today contribute in some way to the health and happiness of [this person]." It doesn't matter whether there is any logical link between your actions and this person's well-being. Simply making this dedication will inspire your own courage and strengthen your connection to this person.

Bring to mind someone who has experienced great challenges or suffering. Imagine the courage it took for this person to face these experiences. Allow yourself to feel, in your body, what you imagine this courage feels like or your own sense of admiration for this person. Realize that this person, like all other people, is not unique in his or her courage. You, too, have the strength to handle extraordinary as well as ordinary challenges. Repeat in your own mind, "Just like me, this person experiences fear. Just like me, [he or she] has doubts. And just like [him or her], I can face today with courage and willingness."

Bring to mind the memory of a time you acted with courage or a time when you experienced the satisfaction of doing something difficult. As you think about this time, remember how it felt in your body, and see if you can reexperience this feeling now.

When you find a meditation that inspires a sense of hope and courage, commit to a daily practice for at least one week. Plant and nourish the seeds of courage and connection, and observe how the meditation influences you over time.

## Other Citta Bhavana Meditations

You can also create your own meditations for any state of mind that you would like to cultivate. Simply follow the two principles of citta bhavana: (1) bring to mind specific words or thoughts that reflect this state of mind, the memory of a time you authentically felt this way, or someone/something that naturally inspires this state of mind in you, and (2) focus on the feeling-state that goes along with these thoughts, memories, and visualizations.

## Reactions to Citta Bhavana

Although citta bhavana meditations are some of the most healing tools in all of yoga, for many people they feel the least natural at first. If you feel like you're faking the emotion or just going through the motions, don't worry, and don't assume that the meditation is not working.

Citta bhavana meditations are a bit like gardening. The first time you try a meditation, you plant the seed of the positive emotion. Each time you return to the meditation, you are watering the seed, creating a nurturing environment for it to grow in. You may not see the results right away, even as the seed is growing. But with time and consistent care, the seed takes strong root, and the plant emerges from the earth.

This is how citta bhavana meditations work. At some point, the seed takes root in your mind and expresses itself in your thoughts, emotions, and actions. So do not worry if these meditations feel unnatural at first. Plant the seed, nurture it, and wait to see what develops.

# PRATIPAKSHA BHAVANA (MOVING THE MIND IN THE OPPOSITE DIRECTION): A MEDITATION TECHNIQUE FOR PAIN AND DIFFICULT EMOTIONS

*Notice (or imagine) one sensation, emotion, or thought and then consciously shift your attention to its opposite. Shift back and forth several times, developing your ability to welcome all experiences but also choose the focus of your experience in the present moment.*

*Practice:*

- *Anytime to develop emotional resilience and the skill to transform pain and suffering.*

- *During stress, pain, or other difficult emotional episodes.*

- *For as long as desired or needed.*

Pratipaksha bhavana meditation demonstrates and strengthens the power of your attention and imagination to determine your experience. The purpose of this meditation is to help you discover that your mind is a safe place. You have the inner strength to handle whatever comes up, and you are not at the mercy of your thoughts and emotions.

This is a challenging practice; you should approach it in small steps, gradually increasing your comfort and confidence with this meditation. Regularly practicing shamatha (befriending the mind) will provide a strong foundation for this meditation.

Pratipaksha bhavana begins with a protective technique that builds your ability to transform thoughts, sensations, and emotions. The second part is a therapeutic technique to use when you are experiencing pain and difficult emotions. However, it is very important to practice the protective technique when you aren't at your lowest low. Develop comfort and skill with the meditation before you need it most, so that you aren't trying to learn it for the first time while you are in more serious pain and suffering.

## The Protective Practice: Exploring Opposites

Practice this form of pratipaksha bhavana meditation when you are not experiencing any particularly strong emotions or sensations but you want to build your capacity to transform pain and suffering.

In any comfortable seated or resting pose, take a few minutes to relax physically and follow your breath. When you are ready, begin to focus your attention on feeling (or imagining) any of the following pairs of opposite states of body and mind. Remember that you are in complete control of this practice. You can choose which pairs of opposites to explore and which you would rather skip. You can at any time change the focus of the meditation.

133

## opposite sensations of the body

- lightness/heaviness
- stillness/movement
- warmth/coolness
- discomfort/comfort
- tension/relaxation

Choose a pair to start with. For the first state in the pair, ask yourself, "Is there anywhere in my body that currently feels this state? What does it feel like? Where do I feel it?" If that state is not currently present, bring to mind a memory of that feeling. Recall what it feels like—the sensations, thoughts, and emotions. After feeling this state, switch to the opposite state and do the same. Then switch back to the first state, feel it again, and switch to the second state, feeling it again. You can switch back and forth as many times as you like. You may even notice that it is possible to feel a pair of opposites at the same time. Finish each pair of opposites either by letting go of both states or by choosing one to rest in before you move on to the next pair.

After you have explored as many opposites as you care to, simply rest with an awareness of your body, without trying to control your attention or experience. Notice how the body feels in this moment and what your mind is naturally drawn to. You can end the practice here or move on to opposites of the mind.

Working with opposite sensations in the body is particularly helpful for working with physical pain. With practice, you will train the mind to focus on other sensations when pain is present.

## opposite states of mind

When it comes to opposites of mind, one opposite in any pair tends to be much more pleasant than its partner. In most of your everyday life, you probably try to avoid the unpleasant states. And yet they pop up anyway, uninvited. It can seem foolish, or even scary, to welcome these thoughts and feelings on purpose. But we do this all the time—just without conscious awareness. Whenever you let the mind wander to the past or future, you create powerful, real emotions that have nothing to do with what is actually happening in the moment. If you let yourself be pulled this way and that by every fleeting thought, your mind can feel more like a minefield than a safe place.

The practice of consciously exploring different states of mind can teach you how not to be afraid of them or overcome by them. You can get to know them as the fleeting impressions they are—things that move through you but that do not define you or control you. As you practice moving between opposites, you will get to know your inner wisdom, the part of yourself that can observe and guide the mind.

- calm/stress
- happiness/sadness
- gratitude/anger
- hope/disappointment

- love/loneliness
- courage/fear
- self-confidence/self-criticism

Start with the pair that seems least intimidating to you. For each state in the pair, ask yourself first: "Is this state present now? Am I feeling it anywhere in my mind and body?" If it is present, ask yourself what it feels like. If not, bring to mind either a memory of a time when you felt this way or simply the memory of how this state feels. As you bring these memories to mind, notice how this state of mind feels in your body.

After a few moments, switch to the opposite state and go through the process again. Are you feeling this state anywhere now, in body or mind? Can you remember a time when you felt that way? Be gentle with yourself as you shift your mind to the "unpleasant" opposite and remember that you can switch back to its healing opposite at any time.

If you choose to remember a time when you felt this way, try not to get lost in thoughts about what happened and why you felt this way. Just use the memory to trigger the feeling, and then drop the story and invite in the feeling-state of it. If you find yourself getting stuck on the story, remember the practice of shamatha (befriending the mind). Bring your awareness to how it feels to breathe in and breathe out, and let the thoughts go.

After you have explored the less pleasant opposite, switch back to the more pleasant state of mind. Notice if one opposite feels stickier, or harder to shift away from, than the other. With focus and practice, you will be able to more easily and quickly change your state of mind and body. Rest in the feeling of the "positive" state for a few moments, allowing yourself to feel it in your body. Finish by coming back to the feeling of your body and breath exactly as it is in this moment.

After you have explored as many opposites as you care to (and often, one pair is enough!), simply rest with an awareness of your body and mind. Do not try to control your attention or experience. Notice how your body feels in this moment and what your mind is naturally drawn to. Notice any observations and insights you have about yourself from this practice. If this meditation brought up strong memories, emotions, or insights, it can be helpful to take some time to write about them or even share your experience with someone you trust.

## The Transformational Practice: Choosing Healing

Use this form of pratipaksha bhavana meditation during times of pain and difficult emotions.

Begin in any position that makes you feel more comfortable, safe, or cared for. See chapter 6 for some possible relaxation poses.

### being present with the physical or emotional pain

An important part of this practice is first allowing yourself to feel the state of mind and body that you want to transform. Transformation is not the same thing as suppression. If you try to block out what you are feeling, it will likely grow stronger. So start where you are. What is happening in your mind and body right now? Notice any sensations, thoughts, or emotions, including those that are causing you pain and suffering. Watch these sensations, thoughts, and emotions come and go in the body and mind, much like you might watch the sensations of the breath as it enters and exits the body.

Create a safe container for whatever it is you are feeling. This doesn't mean you need to get caught up in the story of the emotion—thinking about why you feel this way or what it means. Instead, stay with your body and breath and just notice what this pain or emotion feels like. There is no set amount of time you need to do this: ten breaths might be long enough; at other times, ten minutes might be appropriate. You are looking for a sense of acceptance, even welcoming, what you are feeling. When you feel like you are no longer resisting or trying to block it out, you are ready for the next stage.

### choosing an opposite

Ask yourself, "If I were completely free of this [pain, stress, fatigue, anger, fear, etc.], what would I be feeling or thinking instead? What state of mind and body would heal what I am feeling right now?" The answer (be it comfort, healing warmth, energy, acceptance, forgiveness, gratitude, courage, and so on) will become the focus of your meditation. You can choose more than one opposite to explore, but focus on one at a time.

### creating the opposite

Bring to mind a memory of how your opposite state feels. You can bring to mind a specific memory of when you felt this way, or you can simply bring to mind the memory of how it feels. If there is an image, a person, a mantra, or anything else that naturally inspires this feeling in you, you can focus on that. Allow yourself to feel the body sensations that go along with this state of mind and feel it washing over mind and body. Stay with this process as long as you like.

### welcoming opposites

To end the meditation, let your attention come back to how you feel in this moment. Let go of any attempt to control what you are thinking or feeling. Simply notice what is present for you in this moment. You may find that you are feeling calmer and more relaxed. You may find that one of your two opposites returns. Do not force or resist any thoughts or feelings. Finish this meditation by acknowledging to yourself that you have the strength to handle all sensations, thoughts, and emotions and the freedom to choose healing.

## Jim's Story: The Opposite of Pain

Jim, a U.S. Army veteran who had recently returned from Iraq, had lost his left arm in a roadside explosion. Two months after his amputation surgery, he occasionally had the sense that his left arm was still a part of his body. Unfortunately, he didn't feel any sense of control over the arm. When the phantom arm came into his awareness, it felt tense and uncomfortably stiff. Soon the tension became painful, like a muscle cramp, and was accompanied by a throbbing heat.

Jim was in an intensive rehabilitation program to help him with the transition back to civilian life. As part of this program, he was learning visualization techniques for coping with his phantom arm pain. One technique used the principle of opposites, much like pratipaksha bhavana meditation does.

Jim was taught to use the pain-free sensations of his right arm as an opposite of his phantom left arm pain. When his phantom arm came into awareness, he focused his attention on the sensations of relaxation and coolness in his right arm. Then, as he focused on these sensations in his right arm, he imagined his phantom limb unclenching and relaxing. Next, he moved his right arm and focused on the feelings of lightness and ease as he moved it. Then, as he moved his right arm, he imagined his phantom arm moving with ease. He finished by imagining that he could stretch his phantom limb and then relax it by his side, fist unclenched and muscles free of tension.

This meditation usually led to a helpful decrease in the pain intensity of his phantom limb, and over the course of a few months, Jim was mostly free of the phantom pain.

Meditation techniques like this are currently being explored in many clinical settings, not just with phantom limb pain but with many forms of chronic pain. Researchers are discovering that imagination is a powerful tool for healing pain and can lead to real changes in how the brain processes pain (MacIver et al. 2008).

When you are in pain, what is an opposite sensation that you can focus on? Can you imagine these sensations spreading to the part of your body that is in pain? A technique like this can take time to learn, but if you have an open mind, you may find that imagination can lead to real transformation.

## putting it together

You're now ready to create your own personal yoga program. You have learned all the tools you need to build a healing yoga practice that fits your life and supports your body, mind, and spirit. The next chapter will show you how to put together your favorite practices for befriending the body, breathing, movement, relaxation, and meditation.

# Chapter 8

# your personal yoga program

Personalizing your yoga practice is the best way to make sure that it gives you the experience of health and well-being. This chapter will help you put together a personal yoga program that includes four different types of practices:

1.  A homecoming practice that you can do in just a few minutes to reconnect to mind, body, and spirit.

2.  A yoga ritual to start or end your day with.

3.  A longer protective practice, to develop vitality, resilience, wisdom, and joy.

4.  A healing therapeutic practice for when you are in physical pain, exhausted, or emotionally overwhelmed.

You may find that one of these types of practice works better in your life than others and choose to stick with that one practice. Or you may decide to make them all a part of your life. Yoga doesn't have to take a long time or be done the same way every day. Some days you'll want a very short practice, and other days you'll have the time to spend thirty minutes or more. Some days you'll feel strong, and some days you'll need something gentle. These four types of practices give you a lot of options, so you can always choose a practice that meets your needs.

For each practice type, you'll find sample practices to follow, as well as guidelines for creating your own practices. You may be reluctant to trust your own judgment in putting together a yoga practice. My students often tell me that they feel like they don't know enough about yoga to create a personal yoga program and want to be given the one "right" practice. If you feel this way, you can start by following the sample practices. As you explore the different practices, you'll soon see that there is no one right way or one magic formula. Trust your body and your inner wisdom. Be willing to create a yoga practice the world has never seen before—but is just perfect for you.

# the homecoming practice ("instant" yoga)

A homecoming practice is one simple yoga practice that helps you reunite with body, mind, and spirit. It should be something that brings you home to your body and breath in this moment and helps you let go of stress, pain, and suffering. Your homecoming practice should be something that makes you feel better immediately. It should take only a few minutes at most and be something you can do almost anywhere without fanfare or fuss. It can be any yoga practice you've learned in this book, or it can be your own unique spin on something you've learned. The most important thing is that it has to be something you will actually use throughout the day, whenever you need it.

## Creating a Homecoming Practice

Here are some ideas for practices that will help you reconnect to your mind, body, and spirit:

- Hands-on Breath Awareness (p. 26)

- The Breath of Joy (p. 40)

- The Sun Breath (p. 80)

- Relaxation in Supported Inversion (p. 106)

- Shamatha (Befriending the Mind) Meditation (p. 123)

- Mantra Meditation with favorite mantra (p. 126)

- One phrase from your favorite meditation or check-in question from your favorite reflection, such as "I am already whole and already healed," or "Is there anything I should know?"

## Choosing Your Homecoming Practice

Is it really that important to pick just one practice? Yes. Part of what makes a homecoming practice healing is the intention and energy you give it over time. This takes commitment and consistency. The more you "come home" to this practice, the more it will become a source of comfort. With time, the mind and body will learn to associate this practice with relaxation, pain relief, and peace of mind. The benefits of the practice will then become even stronger and more immediate.

Choosing just one practice will make it much more likely that you will remember to use it. If you have lots of options that you've only tried once or twice, you may end up taking advantage of none of them when you really need them. But if you have one thing that you know will calm your mind, restore your energy, and remind you of your true nature, you will have the confidence to use it.

The following questions may help you find your homecoming practice:

- What yoga practice gives you the most immediate sense of well-being or peace of mind?

- If you could practice only one thing you learned in this book for the rest of your life, what would it be?

- When during the day do you experience the greatest stress or pain? Consider what you are likely to be doing and where you are likely to be. What yoga practice could you reasonably do at these times?

- Do you feel most at home when you reconnect to your body, your mind, your breath, or your inner wisdom and joy? What is the simplest practice you have that reconnects you to this?

- Go back through each of the practice chapters of this book, starting with the breathing practices in chapter 3. Skim through the instructions and remind yourself of everything you have tried or meant to get around to trying. What stands out for you in each chapter? What is most appealing? In each chapter, star the practice that instinctively catches your attention. What is the simplest version of this practice?

- Center yourself with a few minutes of relaxation, breath awareness, or meditation. Then ask yourself, "What is my homecoming practice?" Trust your inner wisdom.

If you came up with several ideas, take a week to try each one out as a homecoming practice for one day. Ask yourself how well it works in your life. Did you remember to use it? If so, how did it make you feel? At the end of the day, how did you feel?

Once you have chosen a homecoming practice, commit to practicing it at least once a day. This will strengthen your connection to it and make it a more powerful personal practice. You might make it your first-thing-when-waking morning ritual or part of your going-to-bed routine. You might choose external cues to remind you (such as the beep of your watch each hour, every time you check email, or before every meal). Whatever you decide to try, make your homecoming practice a regular part of your life.

# the yoga ritual

There is something intrinsically healing about ritual. When you make yoga a daily ritual, it can provide a sense of purpose, stability, and meaning in your life. A yoga ritual can be practiced in the morning, as a way of setting your intention for the day, or in the evening, as a way of undoing any of the stress of the day and preparing for restorative sleep.

A yoga ritual is more formal than the instant yoga of a homecoming practice, but it should still be simple and short enough (say, fifteen minutes or less) that you're not likely to talk yourself out of it. Most importantly, a yoga ritual should remind you of your personal reasons for practicing yoga. The right yoga ritual for you will recommit you each day to healing your mind and body and living life with joy and courage.

Throughout this book, you've read the stories of many people who use yoga to handle everyday stress and pain. Many of these stories featured yoga rituals:

*Jason's story (chapter 4):* To commit to finding more balance in his life, Jason made seated morning meditation a daily ritual.

*Greg's story (chapter 5):* To reduce muscle stiffness and manage his knee and back pain, Greg developed a fifteen-minute movement practice to do every day after work.

*Megan's story (chapter 6):* To help her cope with anxiety, Megan made conscious relaxation a regular part of her life, especially when she was in pain.

*Louisa's story (chapter 4):* To practice befriending her body, Louisa practiced the compassion meditation daily and kept a body gratitude list by her bed. She made a ritual of adding one thing to it each night before she went to sleep.

*Ann's story (chapter 3):* To overcome insomnia, Ann used the breath-freeing chair stretches before going to bed and breath visualizations in bed to help her fall asleep each night.

## Creating Your Own Morning Yoga Ritual

The following ideas may help you come up with your own yoga ritual to practice each morning.

Connecting to your breath and body will give you more energy and enthusiasm to face the day. Choose your favorite breathing exercise and follow it with one or more of your favorite two-pose flows from chapter 5.

Shamatha (befriending the mind) is a perfect meditation practice for first thing in the morning. The clarity and focus you develop will carry into the rest of the day, helping you make conscious choices that support your health and well-being.

Citta bhavana meditations are an excellent way to set your intention for the day. What you choose to focus on first thing can influence how you experience the rest of your day. Which of these meditations appealed most to you? Choose one of these meditations and make it your morning ritual, in or out of bed.

Take one thing you already do every morning—shower, make coffee, cook—and add your favorite mantra meditation to it.

## Creating Your Own Evening Yoga Rituals

The following ideas may inspire your own evening yoga ritual.

Relaxation helps to unravel the stress of the day and prepare you for a good night's sleep. Choose one or more of your favorite restorative yoga poses and add any meditation or breathing practice that brings you peace of mind.

The evening is an excellent time to befriend your body. Which of the reflections or meditations in chapter 4 appealed the most to you? Make a ritual of journaling about one of these reflections, or practicing one of these meditations, each night.

Plenty of yoga practices can be done in bed, and many of them will make it easier to fall asleep. Some of the best pre-sleep practices are the relief breath, breathing the body, conscious relaxation, mantra meditation, citta bhavana meditations, and the pratipaksha bhavana meditation on finding opposites in the body.

Here are some other questions to help you find your yoga rituals:

- Why did you choose to begin a yoga practice? What is the intention for your practice? Of all the practices you've learned in this book, which one helps the most or best reflects this intention?

- Of the practices you've tried in each chapter, which provides you with the greatest sense of hope? Which provides you with the greatest sense of energy? Try any one of these practices, or put them together, as a morning ritual.

- Which of the practices in this book provides you with the greatest sense of relaxation and peace? Which provides you with the greatest relief from pain or stress? Try these practices as an evening ritual.

- What practice gives you the greatest sense of connecting to your inner wisdom—the ability to be a guide for your mind, listen to your body, and choose an experience of peace? Try this practice as a morning or evening ritual.

- What practice gives you the greatest sense of connecting to your natural joy—the sense of gratitude, willingness to face life, and being connected to something bigger? Try this practice as a morning or evening ritual.

- Center yourself with a few minutes of relaxation, breath awareness, or meditation. Then ask yourself, "What is my yoga ritual?" Trust your inner wisdom.

You may find it helpful to record your morning and evening rituals. If you like, you can use the following blank pages to describe your own personal rituals.

# your morning yoga ritual

A daily morning yoga ritual can provide a sense of purpose, stability, and meaning in your life. Use this page to design your practice or record your thoughts about how your practice influences your body, mind, and spirit.

*Only when a yoga practice is followed for a long time, with joy and enthusiasm, will its full benefits be known.*

—Patanjali's *Yoga Sutra*, second century CE

145

## your evening yoga ritual

An evening yoga ritual is a wonderful way to end the day with an act of self-care and healing. Use this page to design your practice or record your thoughts about how your practice influences your body, mind, and spirit.

_The attainment of perfect wisdom and freedom from suffering is a gradual process._

—Patanjali's _Yoga Sutra_, second century CE

# the protective practice

The protective practice is a longer, well-balanced yoga practice that deepens your connection to mind, body, and spirit. It should include a balance of breath, movement, relaxation, and meditation. A well-balanced longer yoga practice will build your resilience and capacity for healing, protecting you from future pain and suffering. It will build your strength and range of motion, increase body awareness, free your natural breath, lift your mood, and contribute to long-term improvements in physical and emotional well-being. You may not have time to do a longer practice every day, but you should aim for practicing on a regular basis, preferably at least twice a week.

## Sample Protective Practices

You may want to choose from one of the five sample protective practices that follow, or you can create your own, using the worksheet at the end of this section.

## 🌿 the prana flow practice 🌿
### (thirty to fifty minutes)

**Breath:** Freeing the Breath series of stretches with Hands-on Breath Awareness (ten to fifteen minutes).

**Movement** (ten to fifteen minutes):

*The Drawbridge:* Practice five times as a flow. Then hold bridge pose for five breaths, and knees-to-chest pose for five breaths. Add internal repetition of mantra of the breath (*so hum*) in knees-to-chest pose.

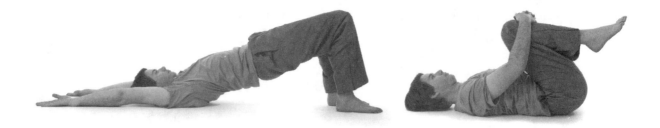

*Cobra Rising:* Practice ten times as a flow. Then hold cobra pose for five breaths and resting cobra for five breaths. Add internal repetition of mantra of the breath (*so hum*) in resting cobra.

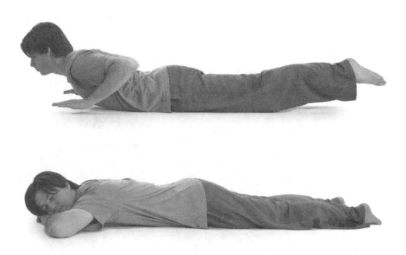

*Bowing in Gratitude:* Practice five times as a flow. Then hold downward-facing dog pose for five breaths and child's pose for five breaths. Add internal repetition of mantra of the breath (*so hum*) in child's pose.

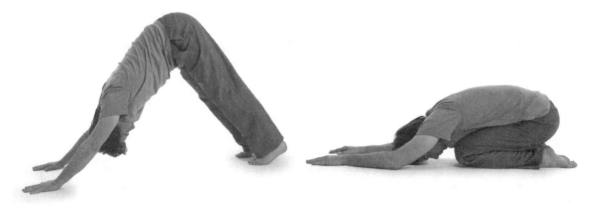

Relaxation: Supported backbending pose (two to five minutes), supported forward bend (two to five minutes).

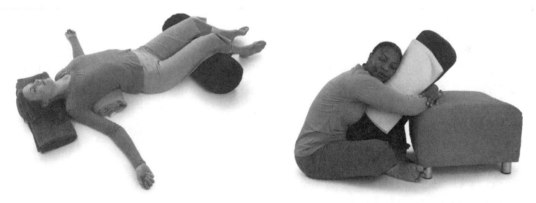

Breath meditation: Breathing the Body in relaxation pose (five to ten minutes).

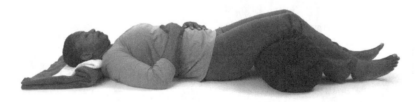

a practice for choosing peace
(thirty to forty minutes)

**Breath/meditation:** Hands-on Breath Awareness in any comfortable seated or relaxation pose. End with internal repetition of the mantra for peace, *om shanti om* (five minutes).

**Movement** (fifteen to twenty minutes): This sequence has a calming effect enhanced by holding the resting pose of each flow after you practice the flow.

*Sun Breath:* Practice five times as a flow. Then hold mountain pose for five breaths. On the last exhalation, repeat "om shanti om" internally or out loud.

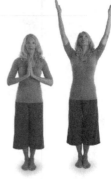

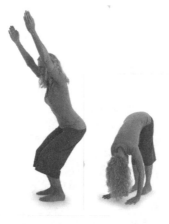

*Strength and Surrender:* Practice five times as a flow. Then hold forward fold for five breaths. On the last exhalation, repeat "om shanti om" internally or out loud.

*Bowing in Gratitude:* Practice five times as a flow. Then hold child's pose for five breaths. On the last exhalation, repeat "om shanti om" internally or out loud.

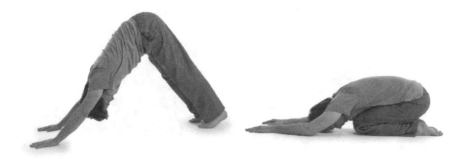

*The Drawbridge:* Practice five times as a flow. Then hold knees-to-chest pose for five breaths. On the last exhalation, repeat "om shanti om" internally or out loud.

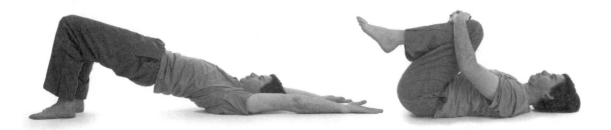

*Resting Twist:* Ten breaths each side. On the last exhalation on each side, repeat "om shanti om" internally or out loud.

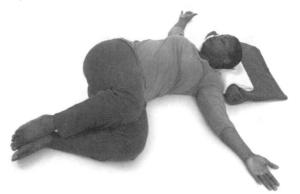

**Relaxation:** Rest in Supported Inversion (five minutes).

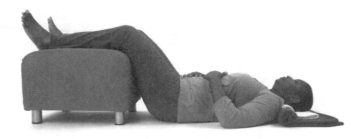

**Meditation:** Shamatha (befriending the mind) in any comfortable seated position (five to ten minutes).

a practice for courage and connection
(thirty to forty minutes)

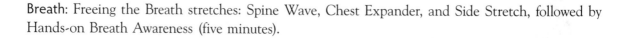

**Breath**: Freeing the Breath stretches: Spine Wave, Chest Expander, and Side Stretch, followed by Hands-on Breath Awareness (five minutes).

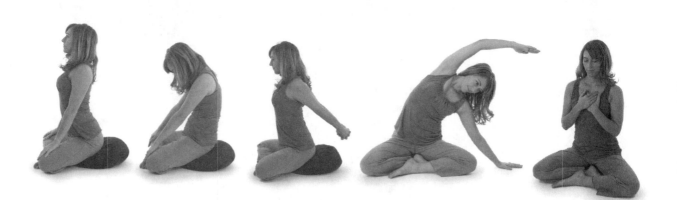

**Meditation**: Dedicate practice to someone you care for or someone who needs support and encouragement (one to two minutes).

**Movement** (all poses held rather than connected as flows; fifteen minutes):

Mountain Pose, five breaths

Sun Pose, ten breaths

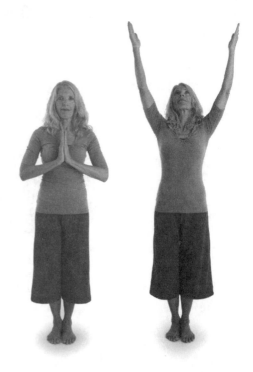

Right side: Peaceful Warrior Pose, five breaths; Courageous Warrior Pose, ten breaths

Left side: Peaceful Warrior Pose, five breaths; Courageous Warrior Pose, ten breaths

Mountain Pose, five breaths

Fierce Pose, ten breaths

Forward Fold, five breaths

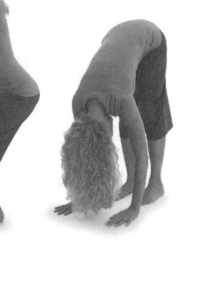

Resting Cobra, five breaths

Cobra Rising, ten breaths

Child's Pose, ten breaths

**Relaxation/meditation** (ten to fifteen minutes):

Supported Bound Angle Pose with any citta bhavana meditation for connection and courage (five minutes).

Rest in Relaxation Pose (five to ten minutes).

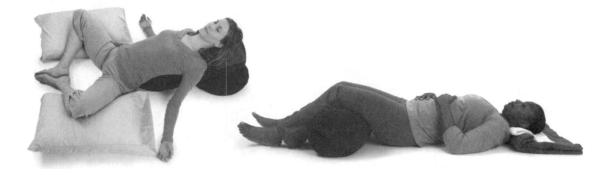

befriending the body and mind
(forty to forty-five minutes)

**Breath:** The Breath of Joy, followed by Compassion Meditation for the Body, Mind, and Spirit (five to ten minutes).

**Movement/relaxation:** Full restorative yoga sequence, five minutes in each pose (thirty minutes):

Supported Inversion

Nesting Pose, right side

Supported Bound Angle Pose

Nesting Pose, left side

Supported Backbending Pose

Supported Forward Bend

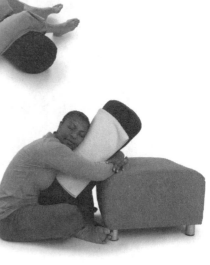

**Meditation:** Shamatha (befriending the mind) in any comfortable seated position, followed by the Listening to Your Body reflection "What do you need?" (five minutes).

## finding balance
## (fifty to sixty minutes)

**Breath:** The Balancing Breath, part 1 (alternate nostril breathing) (five minutes).

**Meditation:** Shamatha (befriending the mind) in any comfortable seated position (five to ten minutes).

**Movement:** Full movement sequence as shown in chapter 5 (thirty minutes):

Sun Breath (five times as flow, and each pose held five breaths)

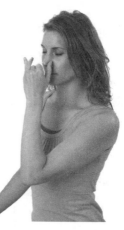

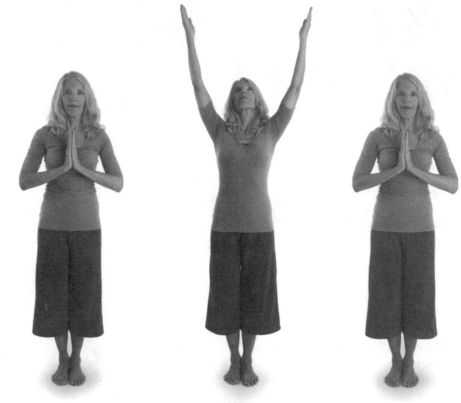

The Yoga Warrior (five times as flow, and each pose held five breaths, both sides)

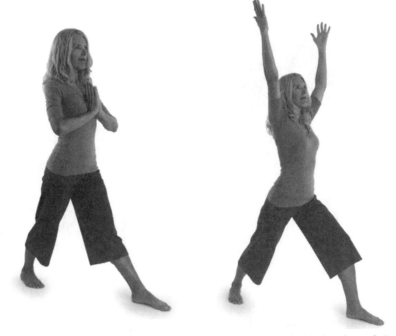

Strength and Surrender (five times as flow, and each pose held five breaths)

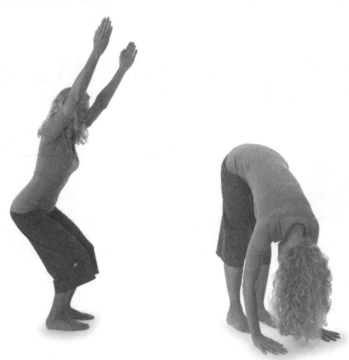

Bowing in Gratitude (five times as flow, and each pose held five breaths)

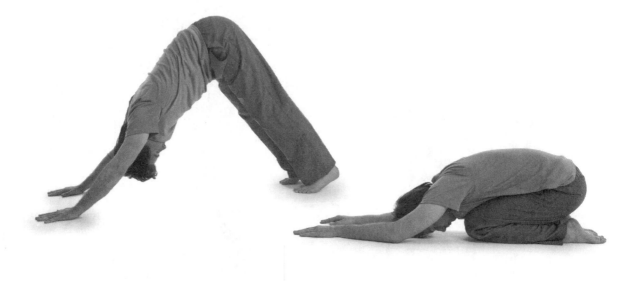

Cobra Rising (five times as flow, and each pose held five breaths)

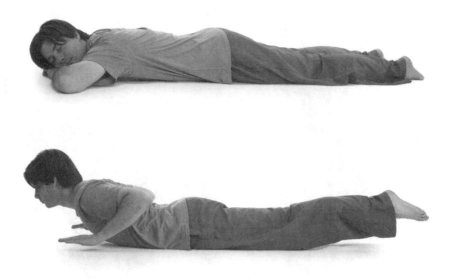

The Drawbridge (five times as flow, and each pose held five breaths)

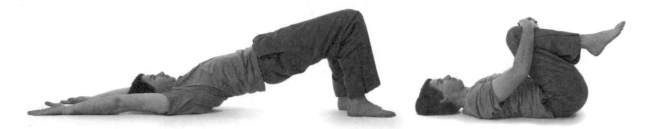

Sweet Dreams (each pose held five breaths on each side)

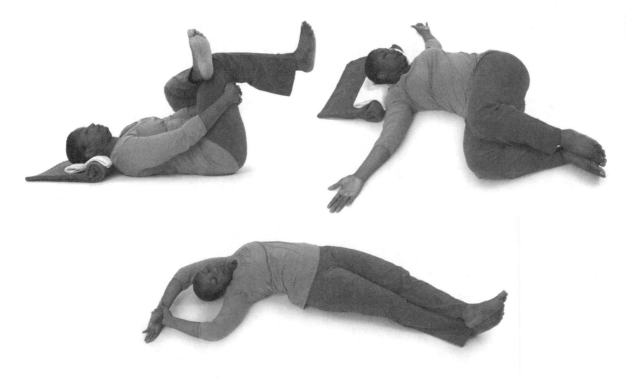

Meditation/relaxation (ten minutes):

Pratipaksha bhavana protective practice in relaxation pose

The Balancing Breath, part 2 (visualization) in relaxation pose

---

# your protective practice

Use this space to design a protective practice for yourself. You may want to make copies of this worksheet so that you can modify your practice or create many practices to meet your different needs and moods.

Theme/name: What is the focus of this practice?

.................................................................................................................................

.................................................................................................................................

Opening breathing/meditation practice:

.................................................................................................................................

.................................................................................................................................

Movement sequence:

.................................................................................................................................

.................................................................................................................................

Closing meditation/relaxation/breathing practice:

.................................................................................................................................

.................................................................................................................................

Notes about this practice: How did this practice make you feel? Did any important thoughts or insights come up during the practice? Each time you practice, take a few moments to record your observations and ideas for future practices.

.................................................................................................................................

.................................................................................................................................

.................................................................................................................................

.................................................................................................................................

.................................................................................................................................

---

# the therapeutic practice

It is important to know that you have something to turn to when you are feeling overwhelmed, exhausted, or in more pain than usual. A therapeutic practice should nurture you, care for you, and relieve stress and pain. It's not the yoga you think you "should" do, but the yoga your body and mind are instinctively drawn to when you are in pain.

Therapeutic practices can be as short or as long as you like. Unlike the longer protective practices, they do not need to be well-rounded with a balance of breathing, movement, relaxation, and meditation practices. A therapeutic practice just needs to support you.

When designing your own therapeutic practice, keep in mind what you are likely to feel up for in difficult times. The practice needs to be so inviting and so unintimidating that you look forward to practicing it even when you are overwhelmed, exhausted, or in pain. Choose an opening breathing, relaxation, or meditation practice that is likely to interrupt the pain or stress response, and stay with it as long as you like. Move on to the rest of the practice when and if you're ready.

## Sample Therapeutic Practices

You may want to try one of the following five therapeutic practices, or create one of you own, using the worksheet at the end of this chapter.

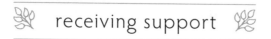

## receiving support

Hold each pose as long as desired:

Supported Inversion with breath awareness

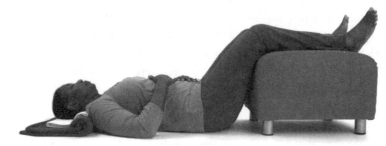

Supported Forward Bend

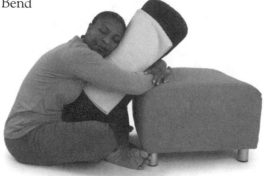

Supported Bound Angle Pose with gratitude reflection

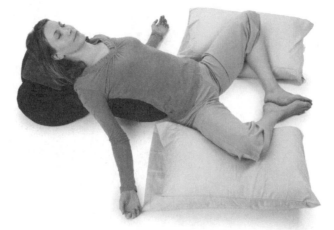

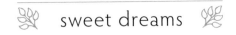

## sweet dreams

Rest in Relaxation Pose with breath awareness (as long as desired).

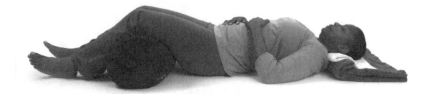

Sweet Dreams movement sequence: Cradle Pose (ten breaths each side); Resting Twist (ten breaths each side); Half Moon Pose (ten breaths each side).

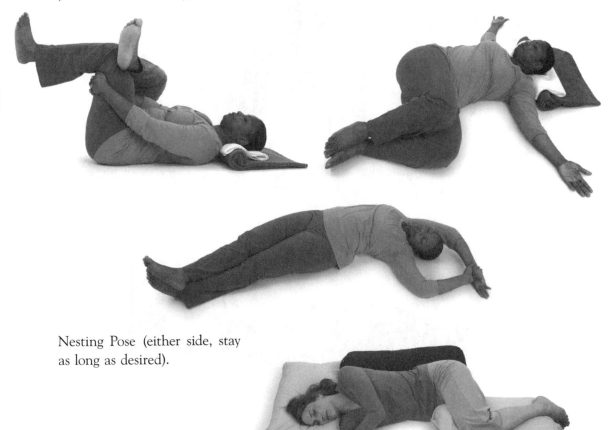

Nesting Pose (either side, stay as long as desired).

### ❧ healing with the breath ❧

Full breath-freeing series of stretches with Hands-on Breath Awareness (see p. 30).

The Breath of Joy (ten breaths).

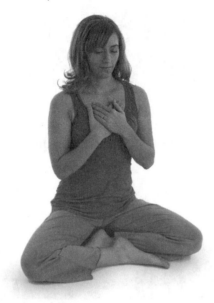

In Relaxation Pose, combine the Body Gratitude meditation with Breathing the Body.

Rest in Relaxation Pose (as long as desired).

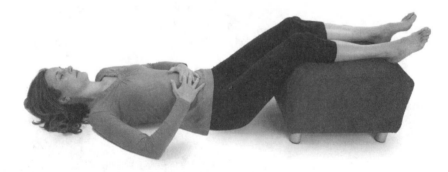

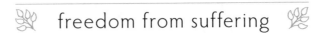

## freedom from suffering

Rest in Relaxation Pose with breath awareness (as long as desired).

The Relief Breath in Relaxation Pose (either counting the breath or using the following internal mantra meditation: "Om" as you inhale, "Om mani padme hum" as you exhale).

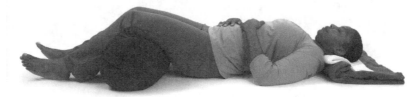

Gentle movement: Knees-to-Chest Pose (ten breaths, then rest for five breaths); Cradle Pose (ten breaths each side, rest for five breaths between sides); seated Side Stretch (ten breaths each side); seated Forward Fold or Child's Pose (ten breaths).

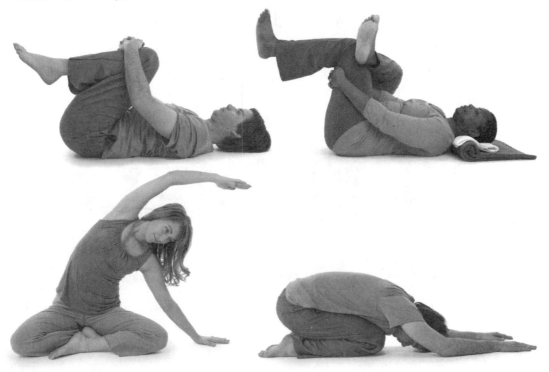

Supported Inversion with meditation on the following phrases: "May I be free of this pain" and "May I be free of suffering."

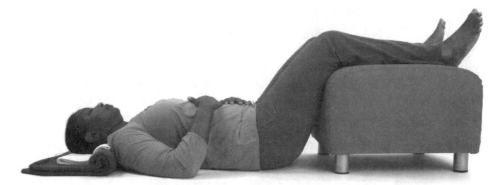

## 🌿 befriending your pain 🌿

Rest in Relaxation Pose with breath awareness (as long as desired).

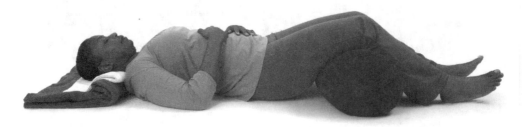

Pratipaksha bhavana therapeutic meditation practice in Relaxation Pose.

Listening to Your Body reflection ("What do you need?" and "Is there anything I should know?").

# your therapeutic practice

Use this space to design a therapeutic practice for yourself. You may want to make copies of this worksheet so you can modify your practice or create many practices to meet your different needs and moods.

Opening: What gentle practice will be inviting and appealing, even when you are in pain, under stress, or low in energy?

Breathing, movement, relaxation, and meditation practices to support healing: What practices make you feel most supported, comfortable, encouraged, and inspired?

Notes about this practice: How did this practice make you feel? Did any important thoughts or insights come up during the practice? Each time you practice, take a few moments to record your observations and ideas for future practices.

# resources

The following resources are ones I have personally enjoyed and recommend to my students. I hope they inspire your continued learning and practice.

## meditation and yoga instruction (books)

*Five Good Minutes in Your Body: 100 Mindful Practices to Help You Accept Yourself and Feel at Home in Your Body* by Jeffrey Brantley and Wendy Millstine (New Harbinger Publications, www.new harbinger.com)

*The Gift of Loving-Kindness: 100 Meditations on Compassion, Generosity, and Forgiveness* by Mary Brantley and Tesilya Hanauer (New Harbinger Publications, www.newharbinger.com)

*The Heart of Yoga: Developing a Personal Practice* by T.K.V. Desikachar (Inner Traditions, store.inner traditions.com)

*Nothing Happens Next: Responses to Questions About Meditation* by Cheri Huber (Keep It Simple, www.livingcompassion.org)

*Relax and Renew: Restful Yoga for Stressful Times* by Judith Hanson Lasater (Rodmell, www.rodmell press.com)

*Yoga as Medicine: The Yogic Prescription for Health and Healing* by Yoga Journal and Timothy McCall (Random House, www.randomhouse.com)

*Yoga R$_x$: A Step-by-Step Program to Promote Health, Wellness, and Healing for Common Ailments* by Larry Payne and Richard Usatine (Random House, www.randomhouse.com)

## meditation and yoga instruction (audio/dvd)

*Body Awareness and Imagination* CD by Matthew McKay and Patrick Fanning (New Harbinger Publications, www.newharbinger.com)

*Emotional Freedom* CDs by Cheri Huber (Sounds True, www.soundstrue.com)

*The Essential Low Back Program: Relieve Pain and Restore Health* book and CDs by Robin Rothenberg (Pacific Institute of Yoga Therapy, www.essentialyogatherapy.com)

*Gentle Yoga Kit: Nurturing the Body, Soothing the Soul* book and CDs by Stephen Cope (Red Wheel, www.redwheelweiser.com)

*Guided Mindfulness Meditation* CDs by Jon Kabat-Zinn (Center for Mindfulness in Medicine, www.mindfulnesscds.com)

*Healing Yoga for Aches and Pains* DVD with Charles Matkin and Lisa Matkin (Anchor Bay, www.anchorbayentertainment.com)

*How to Meditate: A Practical Guide to Making Friends with Your Mind* CDs by Pema Chödrön (Sounds True, www.soundstrue.com)

*LifeForce Yoga Bhavana: A Guided Relaxation Experience* CD by Amy Weintraub (Lifeforce Yoga, www.yogafordepression.com)

*The Secret Power of Yoga* CDs by Nischala Joy Devi (Pranamaya, www.pranamaya.com)

*Viniyoga Therapy* DVDs with Gary Kraftsow (Pranamaya, www.pranamaya.com)

*Yoga Nidra: The Meditative Heart of Yoga* book and CD by Richard Miller (Sounds True, www.soundstrue.com)

## yoga props for restorative yoga

The following companies provide quality yoga props at discounted prices:

Yoga Accessories, www.yogaaccessories.com (1-888-886-YOGA)

Yoga Direct, www.yogadirect.com (1-800-331-8233)

## music for movement, meditation, and relaxation

Music can inspire your yoga practice and create a healing environment anytime, anywhere. The following labels produce music specifically designed for yoga, meditation, and relaxation. The recommended artists and titles are the ones I use most often in my own practice and classes.

Real Music, www.realmusic.com (415-331-8273). Recommended: Ben Leinbach, Buedi Siebert, Namaste Series.

Sounds True, www.soundstrue.com (1-800-333-9185). Recommended: Krishna Das, Maneesh de Moor, Wah!

Spirit Voyage Records, www.spiritvoyage.com (1-888-735-4800). Recommended: Dave Stringer, Girish, Snatam Kaur.

White Swan Records, www.whiteswanrecords.com (1-800-840-5056). Recommended: Deva Premal, White Swan Yoga Masters Series.

## books for people with pain

*The Chronic Pain Care Workbook* by Michael J. Lewandowski (New Harbinger Publications, www.newharbinger.com)

*Full Catastrophe Living: Using the Wisdom of Your Body and Mind to Face Stress, Pain, and Illness* by Jon Kabat-Zinn (Random House, www.randomhouse.com)

*The Mindfulness Solution to Pain* by Jackie Gardner-Nix with Lucie Costin-Hall (New Harbinger Publications, www.newharbinger.com)

*Suffering Is Optional: Three Keys to Freedom and Joy* by Cheri Huber (Keep It Simple, www.living-compassion.org)

## nonprofit organizations supporting people with pain

The following organizations provide information, support, and advocacy for people with pain and for their families, friends, and caregivers:

American Chronic Pain Association (www.theacpa.org), P.O. Box 850, Rocklin, CA 95677

American Pain Foundation (www.painfoundation.org), 201 North Charles Street, Suite 710, Baltimore, Maryland 21201

National Pain Foundation (www.nationalpainfoundation.org), 300 E. Hampden Avenue, Suite 100, Englewood, CO 80113

## nonprofit organizations supporting research, education, and professional training in yoga and meditation

The Center for Mindfulness in Medicine, Health Care, and Society (www.umassmed.edu/cfm), University of Massachusetts Medical School, 55 Lake Avenue, North Worcester, MA 01655. Supports research and training in mind-body approaches to medicine, including the use of mindfulness for chronic pain.

The International Association of Yoga Therapists (www.iayt.org), 115 S. McCormick Street, Suite 3, Prescott, AZ 86303. Supports yoga therapy research and training and serves as a professional organization for yoga teachers, yoga therapists, and healthcare professionals who use yoga in their practice.

The Mind and Life Institute (www.mindandlife.org), 7007 Winchester Circle, Suite 100, Boulder, CO 80301. Supports research on meditation and coordinates collaboration between leaders in contemplative practices, psychology, neuroscience, education, and medicine.

# references

Arch, J. J., and M. G. Craske. 2006. Mechanisms of mindfulness: Emotion regulation following a focused breathing induction. *Behaviour Research and Therapy* 44:1849–1858.

Benson, Herbert. 1975. *The Relaxation Response.* New York: Morrow.

Bernardi, L., P. Sleight, G. Bandinelli, S. Cencetti, L. Fattorini, J. Wdowczyc-Szulc, and A. Lagi. 2001. Effect of rosary prayer and yoga mantras on autonomic cardiovascular rhythms: Comparative study. *BMJ* 323:1446–1449.

Bormann, J. E., T. L. Smith, S. Becker, M. Gershwin, L. Pada, A. H. Grudzinski, and E. A. Nurmi. 2005. Efficacy of frequent mantram repetition on stress, quality of life, and spiritual well-being in veterans: A pilot study. *Journal of Holistic Nursing* 23:395–414.

Burns, J. W. 2006. Arousal of negative emotions and symptom-specific reactivity in chronic low back pain patients. *Emotion* 6:309–319.

Cahn, B. R., and J. Polich. 2006. Meditation states and traits: EEG, ERP, and neuroimaging studies. *Psychological Bulletin* 132:180–211.

Carson, J. W., F. J. Keefe, T. R. Lynch, K. M. Carson, V. Goli, A. M. Fras, and S. R. Thorp. 2005. Loving-kindness meditation for chronic low back pain: Results from a pilot trial. *Journal of Holistic Nursing* 23:287–304.

Chapman, C. R., R. P. Tuckett, and C. Woo Song. 2008. Pain and stress in a systems perspective: Reciprocal neural, endocrine, and immune interactions. *The Journal of Pain* 9:122–145.

D'Souza, P. J., M. A. Lumley, C. A. Kraft, and J. A. Dooley. 2008. Relaxation training and written emotional disclosure for tension or migraine headaches: A randomized, controlled trial. *Annals of Behavioral Medicine* 36:21–32.

Dietrich, A., and W. F. McDaniel. 2004. Endocannabinoids and exercise. *British Journal of Sports Medicine* 38:536–541.

Eisenberger, N. I., J. M. Jarcho, M. D. Lieberman, and B. D. Naliboff. 2006. An experimental study of shared sensitivity to physical pain and social rejection. *Pain* 126:132–138.

Emmons, R. A., and M. E. McCullough. 2003. Counting blessings versus burdens: An experimental investigation of gratitude and subjective well-being in daily life. *Journal of Personality and Social Psychology* 84:377–389.

Finestone, H. M., A. Alfeeli, and W. A. Fisher. 2008. Stress-induced physiologic changes as a basis for the biopsychosocial model of chronic musculoskeletal pain: A new theory? *The Clinical Journal of Pain* 24:767–775.

Fredrickson, B. L., M. A. Cohn, K. A. Coffey, J. Pek, and S. M. Finkel. 2008. Open hearts build lives: Positive emotions, induced through loving-kindness meditation, build consequential personal resources. *Journal of Personality and Social Psychology* 95:1045–1062.

Garcia-Larrea, L., and M. Magnin. 2008. Pathophysiology of neuropathic pain: Review of experimental models and proposed mechanisms. *Presse Medicale* 37:315–340.

Garfinkel, M. S., A. Singhal, W. A. Katz, D. A. Allan, R. Reshetar, and H. R. Schumacher, Jr. 1998. Yoga-based intervention for carpal tunnel syndrome: A randomized trial. *JAMA: The Journal of the American Medical Association* 280:1601–1603.

Glombiewski, J. A., J. Tersek, and W. Rief. 2008. Muscular reactivity and specificity in chronic back pain patients. *Psychosomatic Medicine* 70:125–131.

Goncalves, L., R. Silva, F. Pinto-Ribeiro, J. M. Pego, J. M. Bessa, A. Pertovaara, N. Sousa, and A. Almeida. 2008. Neuropathic pain is associated with depressive behaviour and induces neuroplasticity in the amygdala of the rat. *Experimental Neurology* 213:48–56.

Gracely, R. H., M. E. Geisser, T. Giesecke, M. A. B. Grant, F. Petzke, D. A. Williams, and D. J. Clauw. 2004. Pain catastrophizing and neural responses to pain among persons with fibromyalgia. *Brain* 127:835–843.

Grant, J. A., and P. Rainville. 2009. Pain sensitivity and analgesic effects of mindful states in zen meditators: A cross-sectional study. *Psychosomatic Medicine* 71:106–114.

Hanley, M. A., K. Raichle, M. Jensen, and D. D. Cardenas. 2008. Pain catastrophizing and beliefs predict changes in pain interference and psychological functioning in persons with spinal cord injury. *The Journal of Pain* 9:863–871.

John, P. J., N. Sharma, C. M. Sharma, and A. Kankane. 2007. Effectiveness of yoga therapy in the treatment of migraine without aura: A randomized controlled trial. *Headache* 47:654–661.

Kabat-Zinn, Jon. 1990. *Full Catastrophe Living*. New York: Dell Publishing.

Kakigi, R., H. Nakata, K. Inui, N. Hiroe, O. Nagata, M. Honda, S. Tanaka, N. Sadato, and M. Kawakami. 2005. Intracerebral pain processing in a yoga master who claims not to feel pain during meditation. *European Journal of Pain* 9:581–589.

Keefer, L., and E. B. Blanchard. 2002. A one year follow-up of relaxation response meditation as a treatment for irritable bowel syndrome. *Behaviour Research and Therapy* 40:541–546.

Kolasinski, S. L., M. Garfinkel, A. G. Tsai, W. Matz, A. Van Dyke, and H. R. Schumacher. 2005. Iyengar yoga for treating symptoms of osteoarthritis of the knees: A pilot study. *Journal of Alternative and Complementary Medicine* 11:689–693.

Lane, J. D., J. E. Seskevich, and C. F. Pieper. 2007. Brief meditation training can improve perceived stress and negative mood. *Alternative Therapies in Health and Medicine* 13:38–44.

Lariviere, W. R., and R. Melzack. 2000. The role of corticotropin-releasing factor in pain and analgesia. *Pain* 84:1–12.

MacIver, K., D. M. Lloyd, S. Kelly, N. Roberts, and T. Nurmikko. 2008. Phantom limb pain, cortical reorganization, and the therapeutic effect of mental imagery. *Brain* 131:2181–2191.

Maihöfner, C., H. O. Handwerker, and F. Birklein. 2006. Functional imaging of allodynia in complex regional pain syndrome. *Neurology* 66:711–717.

McCracken, L. M., and K. E. Vowles. 2008. A prospective analysis of acceptance of pain and values-based action in patients with chronic pain. *Health Psychology* 27:215–220.

Melzack, R. 2001. Pain and the neuromatrix in the brain. *Journal of Dental Education* 65:1378–1382.

Menzies, V., and S. Kim. 2008. Relaxation and guided imagery in Hispanic persons diagnosed with fibromyalgia: A pilot study. *Family and Community Health* 31:204–212.

Montoya, P., W. Larbig, C. Braun, H. Preissl, and N. Birbaumer. 2004. Influence of social support and emotional context on pain processing and magnetic brain responses in fibromyalgia. *Arthritis and Rheumatism* 50:4035–4044.

Morone, N. E., and C. M. Greco. 2007. Mind-body interventions for chronic pain in older adults: A structured review. *Pain Medicine* 8:359–375.

Morone, N. E., C. S. Lynch, C. M. Greco, H. A. Tindle, and D. K. Weiner. 2008. "I felt like a new person." The effects of mindfulness meditation on older adults with chronic pain: Qualitative narrative analysis of diary entries. *The Journal of Pain* 9:841–848.

Orme-Johnson, D. W., R. H. Schneider, Y. D. Son, S. Nidich, and Z. H. Cho. 2006. Neuroimaging of meditation's effect on brain reactivity to pain. *Neuroreport* 17:1359–1363.

Petersen-Felix, S., and M. Curatolo. 2002. Neuroplasticity—an important factor in acute and chronic pain. *Swiss Medical Weekly* 132:273–278.

Philippot, P., G. Chapelle, and S. Blairy. 2002. Respiratory feedback in the generation of emotion. *Cognition and Emotion* 16:605–627.

Porreca, F., M. H. Ossipov, and G. F. Gebhart. 2002. Chronic pain and medullary descending facilitation. *Trends in Neurosciences* 25:319–325.

Riley, J. L. 3rd, C. D. Myers, T. P. Currie, O. Mayoral, R. G. Harris, J. A. Fisher, H. A. Gremillion, and M. E. Robinson. 2007. Self-care behaviors associated with myofascial temporomandibular disorder pain. *Journal of Orofacial Pain* 21:194–202.

Sherman, K. J., D. C. Cherkin, J. Erro, D. L. Miglioretti, and R. A. Deyo. 2005. Comparing yoga, exercise, and a self-care book for chronic low back pain: A randomized, controlled trial. *Annals of Internal Medicine* 143:849–856.

Srivastava, R. D., N. Jain, and A. Singhal. 2005. Influence of alternate nostril breathing on cardio-respiratory and autonomic functions in healthy young adults. *Indian Journal of Physiology and Pharmacology* 49:475–483.

Staud, R., and M. Spaeth. 2008. Psychophysical and neurochemical abnormalities of pain processing in fibromyalgia. *CNS Spectrums* 13:12–17.

Teixeira, M. E. 2008. Meditation as an intervention for chronic pain: An integrative review. *Holistic Nursing Practice* 22:225–234.

Tracey, I., and P. W. Mantyh. 2007. The cerebral signature for pain perception and its modulation. *Neuron* 55:377–391.

Upadhyay Dhungel, K., V. Malhotra, D. Sarkar, and R. Prajapati. 2008. Effect of alternate nostril breathing exercise on cardiorespiratory functions. *Nepal Medical College Journal* 10:25–27.

van Tulder, M. W., B. Koes, and A. Malmivaara. 2006. Outcome of non-invasive treatment modalities on back pain: An evidence-based review. *European Spine Journal* 15 Suppl. 1:S64–S81.

Wu, S. D., and P. C. Lo. 2008. Inward-attention meditation increases parasympathetic activity: A study based on heart rate variability. *Biomedical Research* 29:245–250.

Zhuo, M. 2007. A synaptic model for pain: Long-term potentiation in the anterior cingulate cortex. *Molecules and Cells* 23:259–271.

# index

Kelly McGonigal, Ph.D., is an award-winning instructor at Stanford University, where she teaches yoga, psychology, and healthy back classes. She is a leader in mind-body science and practice, and provides teacher trainings and continuing education for yoga, fitness, and health care professionals. McGonigal is editor-in-chief of the *International Journal of Yoga Therapy* and a frequent writer for publications such as *Yoga Journal* and *IDEA Fitness Journal*.

Visit her online at www.kellymcgonigal.com.

Foreword writer **Timothy McCall, MD**, is a board-certified internist, medical editor of Yoga Journal, and author of two books, *Yoga as Medicine* and *Examining Your Doctor*. He currently lives in the San Francisco Bay area, and presents lectures, seminars, and yoga workshops internationally.

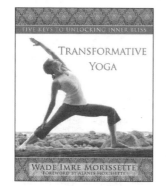
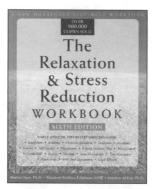
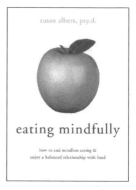
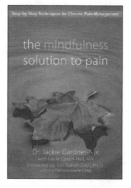
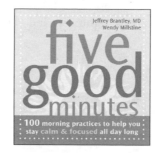
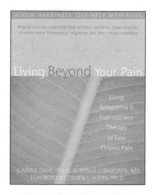